GREAT SEXPECTATIONS

ABOUT THE AUTHORS

Gemma Cribb is a thirty-eight-year-old single woman living in Sydney, Australia who identifies as heterosexual. She is a clinical psychologist with a special interest in sex therapy and relationships. Professionally she has learnt and personally she has explored many theories and expressions of sexuality, including monogamy, polyamory, relationship anarchy, celibacy, sex with people across the gender spectrum, kinky sex, Tantric sex, erotic meditation practices, OMing (orgasmic meditation), as well as great vanilla sex. Gemma has experienced her sexuality in the context of long-term heteronormative relationships as well as in the single-and-dating and non-monogamous worlds.

James Findlay is a thirty-two-year-old single guy living in Melbourne, Australia and identifies as gay. He's a radio producer, writer and broadcaster with a special interest in sex and relationships. This keen interest started in his early twenties when people around the student radio station noticed he was talking about sex and relationships a lot. Before long, he was asked to be a guest on the station's sex and relationships show that he ended up hosting every week not long after. James then went on to co-host and produce the sex programme on Australia's LGBTI radio station, Joy 94.9, before moving on to produce *The Hook Up*, the sex and relationship programme on the national public broadcaster, Triple J. James also holds a Master of Public Health degree, in which he majored in sexual health.

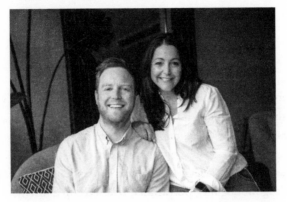

Photo by Jessica Cribb

ALSO BY GEMMA CRIBB

Doing Single Well

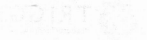

GREAT SEXPECTATIONS

CHANGE YOUR PERSPECTIVE AND HAVE THE SEX YOU REALLY WANT

BY GEMMA CRIBB AND JAMES FINDLAY

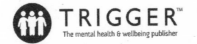

TRIGGER™
The mental health & wellbeing publisher

First published in Great Britain 2020 by Trigger

Trigger is a trading style of Shaw Callaghan Ltd & Shaw
Callaghan 23 USA, INC.

The Foundation Centre

Navigation House, 48 Millgate, Newark

Nottinghamshire NG24 4TS UK

www.triggerpublishing.com

Contributor: James Findlay

British Library Cataloguing in Publication Data

A CIP catalogue record for this book is available upon request
from the British Library

ISBN: 9781789561418

This book is also available in the following e-Book formats:

ePUB: 9781789561425

Cover design by Bookollective

Typeset by Lapiz Digital Services

Printed and bound in Great Britain by CPI Group (UK) Ltd,
Croydon CRO 4YY

DEDICATION

Gemma: Thank you to my teachers, clients and friends who have shared their wisdom, their vulnerabilities and their salacious stories to inspire the writing of this book.

James: Thank you to my mentors and guiding lights who tread this path of sexual enlightenment and education before me. You've not only gifted me with advice and powered me with confidence, but you've allowed me to pass that on to others who'll be able to make their own "great sexpectations" exactly how they want them.

TABLE OF CONTENTS

AUTHORS' NOTE

Writing this book, we wanted to ensure that it was helpful to as many people as possible. Given how heteronormative most books about sex are, we felt it was important to speak in a way that is relatable to people who identify differently to being straight, able-bodied and cisgendered. However, as two able-bodied people, a straight cis-woman and a gay cis-man, we can't possibly have the lived experience nor the authentic voice of someone outside of those parameters (nor can we speak for many inside of those either!). Similarly, neither James nor I pretend to be completely unbiased nor entirely conscious of all the sexpectations that influence us. As such, if your unique experiences aren't adequately covered, we hope that you can still extrapolate from the suggestions we give to improve your understanding of your sex life and sexual preferences.

When the research we cite refers to "women" and "men", you should take this to mean cisgendered women and men – very little of the research we came across allowed for non-binary or non-cisgendered identification. Except for where it doesn't make sense to do so, when we refer to "women" or "female", please assume this means people with a vagina. Similarly, when we refer to "men" or "male", please take this as people with a penis.

We have also included examples of real-life testimonies throughout the book. Most of these quotes have been taken from forums on the internet, from personal conversations with clients, callers (on the radio), and friends. Quotes have been edited for brevity and where permission to reproduce has not been directly granted (e.g. on internet forums), details have been modified to maintain anonymity.

Finally, sex is often not the easiest topic to talk about – hence the existence of this book. But those with experiences of sexual abuse can find the topic especially difficult. Although this book is not about non-consensual sex, it is occasionally referenced or implied and we have tried to flag this ahead of the relevant sections for you to skip if you need to.

Even if you have not had a sexual-abuse history, go gently through this book and check in with your comfort level and feelings along the way. If you find yourself feeling uncomfortable reading a certain section, that section might be a good one to come back to later – or never if your body doesn't consent!

INTRODUCTION

What is sex?

I'll bet the minute you read that question a certain set of images and ideas came to mind, right?

But the interesting question is how did you form that concept of what sex is?

Most of us develop our ideas from a variety of sources and at very early ages, so the answer to that question is often individual and not clearly defined.

In my experience as a sex therapist, we all carry around specific ideas of what sex is, what makes for "good sex", why we have sex, when we should have sex, who it should be with, and what meaning it should have, if any. We all have expectations around sex – sexpectations. And, we rarely question the correctness of these sexpectations, even when they are causing us great distress personally or in our relationships.

Sexpectations are the beliefs that we hold, consciously or unconsciously, about sex. These beliefs are passed down through our cultural upbringing, our family and peer group, and developed through our personal sexual history. They influence our sexual choices and our levels of sexual and relationship satisfaction. Many sexual problems occur largely because of a mismatch between a person's sexpectations and what their or their partner's bodies are able to manage. Understanding and changing your sexpectations to better align with your lived experience of sex can result in an incredible boost to your sexual self-esteem and your experience of sex in your everyday life.

This book is structured loosely into three parts. The first part is an exploration of some sexpectations throughout history, helping you understand just how culturally specific, time specific and changeable sexpectations are. Then we delve into common present-day sexpectations to give you the opportunity to realise which (if any) of these you have absorbed and to contemplate how they might have affected you. Finally, Part 3 will help you strip away your sexpectations and deep dive into a new awareness of your sexual self. You will learn more about your authentic sexuality and how to express it alone or with a partner.

We recommend you go through the book in sequence rather than dipping in and out so that you can understand the full extent of how sexpectations influence us and uncover and work through your own. If there is any terminology you are not familiar with, have a look at the key terms defined overleaf or the glossary at the back of the book.

Throughout the book there are reflective questions and exercises to help you learn about what works and doesn't work for you. They are there to help you apply the concepts we discuss to your own beliefs and experiences so that you can better understand your own sexpectations. Most of the exercises can be done by writing things down, talking about them with a friend or partner, or just thinking the questions over. It could also be useful, if you are in a sexual relationship, to work through the exercises with your partner and compare your responses. *However,* make sure to do them alone first to minimise the risk of you answering to please your partner, save their feelings, or simply to get a sense of where you are at without worrying about what they might think of you.

Through this book we invite you to begin a journey of continual exploration of what type of sexuality and sexual practices you like to engage in and that feel good for your body. We position sex as a neutral activity, much like cooking or exercise, and invite you to join us with curiosity to discover your preferences around sex, just as you would when learning what types of foods you like to eat or sports you like to play. You may find that, deep down, you are not interested in sex, don't want it, or don't want to be good at it, similar to how many people don't like exercise. And that is perfectly fine. This is about *your* journey, and your sexuality.

Our aim is to help you see beyond the sexpectations you have unconsciously absorbed. In doing so, we hope to give you a new lens through which to view yourself and your sexual experiences. Because, only then can you learn the difference between what you *think* you want and what you *really* want. Only then can you make conscious and active choices for your sexual life, instead of defaulting to choices based on what you think sex should be. Ultimately, this process is about becoming an expert in your own sexuality, finding your unique sexual self-expression and staying authentic to it with confidence and security – so you can be your own boss in the bedroom (if that's your thing!).

KEY TERMS

Below is a list of terms that we use in the book and their meaning. At the end of this book you will find a broader glossary of terms for your reference.

Bottoming

Someone who plays the role of receiver and likes having things done to them in a same-sex sexual interaction. The bottom is often the one being penetrated, if penetration occurs.

Cisgendered
A term for people whose gender identity matches the sex that they were assigned at birth.

Heteronormative
The belief that it is normal for people to be one of two distinct and complementary genders (man or woman), be heterosexual, and follow a particular life pathway with specific gender-determined roles (marriage and babies, providers and caregivers, etc.).

Heterosexual
A person who is emotionally, romantically, sexually, affectionately or relationally attracted to members of the opposite sex or gender. Often called a "straight" person.

Homosexual
The clinical term, coined in the field of psychology, for people with a same-sex sexual attraction.

Masturbation
The sexual stimulation of one's own genitals for sexual arousal or sexual pleasure.

Orgasm
The climax of sexual excitement, characterised by intensely pleasurable feelings centred in the genitals. In men it is often experienced as an accompaniment to ejaculation.

Pederasty
Sexual activity involving a man and a pubescent or adolescent boy. This term is primarily used to refer to

historical practices of certain cultures particularly ancient Greece and ancient Rome.

PIA
Abbreviation for "Penis in Anus". Referring to the penetration of an anus by a penis.

PIV
Abbreviation for "Penis in Vagina". Referring to the penetration of a vagina by a penis.

Queer
A term describing people who have a non-normative gender identity, sexual orientation or sexual anatomy. This includes lesbians, gay men, bisexual people, and transgender people.

Sexpectation
The conscious and unconscious beliefs that we hold about sex. These beliefs are learnt through our culture, family, peer group and our personal sexual history. They influence our sexual behaviour and our levels of sexual and relationship satisfaction.

Sexual Energy
The feeling originating generally from the genitals (or in Tantric terms the "sexual chakra") that indicates you are sexually aroused or turned on. It can be experienced differently by different people – heat, tingling, waves of sensation, tension, etc.

PART 1

SETTING THE SCENE FOR OUR SEXPECTATIONS

A Short History of Sex

CHAPTER 1

WHY TALK ABOUT SEXPECTATIONS

At some time in your life (certainly in the English-speaking world) you would have learnt that a cat says "meow" and a dog says "woof". You probably won't remember learning it, and you probably aren't aware that this understanding is now unconscious and automatic in your brain – it has become an expectation. However, if you met a cat that said "quack" or a dog that said "oink", you would quickly become aware that your expectations were not met!

In our daily lives, we are always learning and absorbing information from the world around us, whether consciously or not. In this way, we form expectations about how the world works. When our expectations are not met, we feel confused at best, disappointed, angry and resentful at worst. Repeated disappointment in any area of life can lead to feelings of anxiety, hopelessness, worthlessness and despair. But this is especially so with important or sensitive areas in our lives, where violated expectations throw up stronger feelings of confusion and frustration. Sex is a *very* sensitive area of life for most people! So, whilst we might be mildly perplexed if we met a cat who quacked, most of us would become very distressed if our sex life didn't match our ideas of what we think it should.

It's human nature to blame our problems and distress on other people. Many people blame their sexual partners for their disappointments and frustrations and believe that if only their partner would change, the problem would disappear. A large proportion of the couples I see in therapy begin with this kind of "fix my partner" agenda. However, continued criticism and blame rarely solves the problem and more often leads to disconnection, conflict, and loss of love. Alternatively, if we don't blame someone else for our problems, we tend to blame ourselves. High levels of self-criticism, self-doubt and rumination on our perceived inadequacies is similarly unhelpful for solving problems and resolving distress, and is instead more likely to lead to low self-esteem and depression.

With such serious consequences, it makes sense that we want to be as realistic as possible when setting our expectations, right?

So, how do we form our expectations about sex – our sexpectations?

It is only recently in Western culture that sex was even a topic open for discussion. Traditionally, teenagers have not been given any information on sexual matters because discussion of sex was taboo. Instruction on sex was left to a child's parents and often put off until just before marriage. School-based sex education began in the late nineteenth century, with the first sex education course being run in Britain in 1889. However, much of the focus of sex education in schools centres around the reproductive system, foetal development, and the physical changes of adolescence. The practical, pleasurable, emotional and relationship aspects of sex are often swept under the rug. In fact, it was only in September 2019 that relationship education in primary schools and relationship and sex education in secondary schools was made mandatory in England by the UK government.

Despite these improvements, taboo still clings to the subject of sex. It remains mostly out of sight, with frank and open conversations about this important part of life still feeling too awkward. Because of this lingering taboo and the unhelpful sexpectations we absorb from "informal" sources such as the media and porn, many people feel shame about their sexual desires, sexual function and sex drives (or lack thereof).

Shame results in the avoidance of discussions in this area of our lives. So, our response is, we either elevate or denigrate our ideas of sex. As you can imagine, the elevated "locker-room" stories of sexual prowess and multiple orgasms are not necessarily representative of your friends' actual sexual experiences! Similarly, when we denigrate and complain about our frustration with our partners and our sex lives, we are likewise contributing to the notion that there is a golden standard of sex. This cycle of taboo, shame, secrecy, elevation or denigration self-perpetuates and leaves people accessing and recycling bad information, reinforcing hugely unhelpful sexpectations. We are creators of our own sexual boundaries. And, like quicksand, the more we try to struggle in this way the more stuck we get.

Sex and relationships are important aspects of most people's mental health, wellbeing and self-esteem, but the sources of information at our disposal are inadequate. As a result, most of us have some form of unrealistic or unhelpful sexpectations, with most of the problems I see as a sex therapist due, at least in some part, to these often misguided sexpectations. To release ourselves from this toxic cycle, we need to have a new awareness of what sex is for us as individuals, and this awareness needs to inform new, open and honest conversations around sex.

HOW DID YOU LEARN ABOUT SEX?

'My mum rebelled against her own conservative Catholic upbringing to become a psychologist and sex therapist. As such, I had a fairly non-traditional, sex-positive upbringing. From as early as I can remember, my sister and I would spend Sunday mornings watching TV in our family living room because "Mummy and Daddy were making love". We knew that it was adult time and it was not to be interrupted! I remember talking about sex with my parents from a young age and my mum tells stories of getting called into a parent–teacher interview because primary-school Gemma had been going around telling the other kids that "the clitoris is just for fun!"' – **Gemma**

'Coming from a somewhat conservative upbringing, I've had to forge my own path of sexual exploration. Sex was rarely talked about in our household, but I do remember Mum telling me about how periods worked (no idea why this memory stands out). In high school, I was always the relationship confidant. If a girl had boy problems, we'd walk around the school talking them out. I also remember being up late talking to guys in my year group on MSN Messenger about different masturbation techniques, how big our dicks were, and how far we could blow our loads. I just thought all guys did this, but apparently not.

'I was eighteen when I had my first sexual encounter with a guy. I'd met someone on the internet, and after chatting online for a few weeks, we decided to meet up. He was a thirty-year-old handyman. One night he picked me up in his pickup and he took me to the

local gay sauna. To say it was a bit confronting would be an understatement. There were so many men in towels, naked, playing with each other, having a great time. I didn't touch another guy for a few months after that, but when I eventually hooked up with someone I felt I had a connection with, I knew for sure that was what I was missing from my life. Sex with men.' – **James**

EXERCISE: THE BIRDS AND THE BEES

Think about how you learnt about sex. Were your experiences similar to the above? Below are some questions that will help you begin to unpack your own sexpectations – sexpectations that perhaps you consciously didn't realise you had.

What messages about sex, the explicit (directly told to you) or implicit (in the language used, their feelings about sex, their own sexual behaviours, or in the things that *weren't* said) did you learn from:

- your parents and other adults
- your siblings and peers
- sex education at school
- TV and other media?

Did you learn anything that you later realised was untrue?

What do you wish you had known before you started being sexual?

Think back to your greatest sexual disappointments and frustrations. What caused your dissatisfaction? What sexpectations were not met?

We all had to learn about sex somehow. Whether you feel that you received a good education, or that it was lacking, keep the answers you have generated to the questions above in mind as you read through the rest of the book. They will help you understand how you came to develop the sexpectations you have and give you a point for comparison when you encounter a sexpectation that you *don't* hold.

CHAPTER 2

A HISTORY OF OPPOSITE-SEX SEX

(by Gemma)

Having had basically the same anatomy for around 100,000 years, it is safe to assume that sex has always been pleasurable for us as humans (Buss, 2003). However, whether sex for the sake of pleasure was acceptable or whether sex served another function largely depended on things like culture, era, religion and gender.

Over the course of history there has been a plethora of sexual ideas and practices that have been considered "right" or "wrong" – or maybe more appropriately "socially sanctioned" or not – in society and culture. The following explorations in no way constitute an exhaustive account of different sexpectations throughout the ages. Rather, they serve as a series of examples that illustrate how our sexpectations can be influenced in different ways and how our milieu affects our attitudes towards sex and the role sex plays in our lives and relationships.

RELIGION
Religion has long held a powerful sway over our sexpectations. Most early religions were tolerant of sex

within the context of a marriage, but anything else that didn't lead to procreation was usually viewed as a sin (Shorter, 2005). For example, fornication (sex outside of marriage) is said to have attracted the punishment of one hundred lashes under early forms of traditional sharia (Muslim) law and adultery (Peters, 2012).

Influenced by the stoic philosophers, most notably Augustine, early Christianity saw lust as a deadly sin and viewed nudity as shameful because of its association with humanity's punishment for Adam and Eve's original sin (Tannahill, 2006). Due to this general threat of damnation as a result of pleasure and lust, sexpectations for early Christians considered sex within a marriage preventative (of lust outside the marriage), perfunctory, and with the primary goal of reproduction (Tannahill, 2006). For example, contraception was banned as it removes the reproductive element from the act of sex. It is thought that, between the sixth and sixteenth centuries, some church authorities went as far as to prescribe that intercourse should be face to face, with the man on top (later to be termed the "missionary position" (Kinsey, 1948)) primarily because they believed it led to conception (Priest, 2001). Punishments for those using "deviant" sexual positions could be harsh: up to three years' penance for the woman on top, oral intercourse or sex *a tergo*, the latter of which was seen as the most sinful position, with the possible exception of anal intercourse (Brundage, 1984).

By manner of contrast, in Tantric Buddhism, sex was seen as very spiritual and a pathway to enlightenment; heterosexual sex was a sacred duty, like prayer. To this end, and in stark contrast to sex for procreation, there were teachings on how to stop ejaculation in favour of withholding this "energy" to sublimate it because semen was viewed as a highly potent and spiritually significant substance (Douglas, 1997).

The *Kamasutra*, a well-known text from this philosophy, lists desire, sexuality and emotional fulfilment as some of the proper goals of life. The text contains explicit descriptions of various forms of human sexual activity and positions, explanations on what triggers and sustains desire, and how and when desire is good or bad, as well as when and how to have sex outside of your relationship (Doniger, 2003). As such, the expectations around sex for a Tantric Buddhist would have been radically different to your expectations if you grew up as an early Christian!

GENDER AND LEGITIMACY

Sex hasn't always been as taboo as it is in modern society, with references to sex going as far back as we have historical records (Bell, 1997). The words we have today such as *aphrodisiac*, *eroticism*, *nymphomania* and *homosexuality* are all derived from ancient Greek. The ancient Greek myths of the hero Hercules having ravished fifty virgins in a night and having had an affair with his nephew reveals their relative openness around – almost glorification of – sexuality (Chrystal, 2016). Similarly in Rome, tales of emperors cross-dressing, same-sex sex, prostitution and orgies abound. Roman men could philander as much as they liked so long as their mistress was unmarried, or if their lover was a boy, he was over a certain age. Prostitution was legal, public and widespread (Chrystal, 2017).

Sexpectations for noble women, however, were more conservative. Women were considered the property of men and kept for the purpose of bearing legitimate children. Noble girls were expected to be virgins for their first marriage – which was usually arranged for social or political reasons (Cartwright, 2014). In ancient Rome there is evidence that a woman who had an affair could be punished anywhere along the spectrum of being killed by her husband to him divorcing her and keeping a portion of her dowry (Rawson, 1986). Additionally, whilst it was considered customary for a widow to remain in mourning for ten months before remarrying to allow for the establishment of paternity in any pregnancy, men were not bound by the same formal waiting period (Hersch, 2010).

These gender-specific sexpectations based on ensuring paternity can be seen spanning across cultures. In early China, the virginity of women was rigidly enforced and linked to a woman's monetary value ("bride price"). High-ranking men were expected to take a wife chosen for them by their family but allowed to choose other sexual partners as concubines (Maynes, 1996). Even in the more liberal island of French Polynesia, first-born high-status female children were expected to be chaste whereas other children were initiated into sex as soon as boys were physically able to achieve penetration (Diamond, 2004).

It is for similar reasons that the concept of "courtly love" came into being in the European courts of the late eleventh century. Noble men and women would have been married by their parents for political and financial gain and not for love. Courtly love between a married noblewoman and a troubadour, knight or other man of the courtier class therefore brought romance and sexual passion without the vows of fidelity being broken. Although there is some argument whether this type of love actually existed beyond the literature and storytelling of the time, it can be seen to be the product of the reproductive and successive sexpectations of the time (Newman, 1968).

HEALTH AND MEDICAL UNDERSTANDINGS

When we look at historical health information and medical technology, we get another glimpse into the confusion and conflict that has characterised people's sexpectations for centuries.

In the Middle Ages (fifth to fifteenth century), life was highly influenced by the medical theory of "humours". The humour theory posited that illnesses were caused not by germs, but by an imbalance of essences in the body (Jackson, 2001). Celibacy was considered as equally potentially fatal as sexual overindulgence because both behaviours led to an imbalance of the "seminal" humour. As such, despite sex outside of marriage and masturbation being considered a sin, sex with prostitutes and masturbation for the sake of one's health was condoned by medical authorities to prevent the build-up of the seminal humour (Harvey, 2018).

Because of this, prostitution was considered a necessary evil for unmarried men. However, the threat of acquiring an STD (sexually transmitted disease) was ever present, as was the stigma of them. In medieval times, syphilis and gonorrhoea were two of the most prevalent STDs in Europe (Burg, 2012). The first well-recorded European outbreak of syphilis occurred in 1494 when it broke out amongst French soldiers. As it swept across Europe, it killed over five million people.

Prior to the invention of modern medicines, most notably antibiotics, STDs were generally incurable. In the 18th and 19th centuries, mercury, arsenic and sulphur were commonly used, which often resulted in serious side effects and many people died of mercury poisoning (Burg, 2012). Additionally, the stigma attached often caused a delay in treatment causing the continued transmission of the infection to unsuspecting sexual partners (Harvey, 2018).

It wasn't until 1746, at the London Lock Hospital, that the first treatment for STDs was made available. And, in the second half of the nineteenth century, the Contagious

Diseases Act was passed in order to arrest and treat suspected prostitutes (Walkowitz, 1980).

And what of the effect of medical understandings on female sexuality? In medieval times, regular sexual intercourse was also seen as necessary for women as it was thought that both sexes produced "seed" and if a woman was not sexually active, it would build up and cause suffocation of the womb. Restricted diets, vinegar suppositories and masturbation were thought to relieve the symptoms of this condition, which included fainting and shortness of breath (Harvey, 2018).

Masturbation was not only seen as a treatment for health conditions but was also thought to lessen women's desire for intercourse. Thirteenth-century scholar Albertus Magnus wrote: if women "use their fingers or other instruments until their channels are opened and by the heat of the friction and coition the humour comes out, and with it the heat, their groins are cooled off and they are made more chaste" (as quoted by Harvey, 2018).

In nineteenth-century England, it was deemed a medical fact that if a woman was having trouble conceiving it was because she was not reaching orgasm. Female orgasm therefore became a core sexpectation of the time for reproductive reasons. Female orgasm was also thought to have had further medical benefits with "hysterical paroxysm" (orgasm) being thought of as the cure for "hysteria", a condition which involved symptoms of ongoing anxiety, irritability and a bloated stomach. Because the pelvic massage used to bring about these orgasms was thought to be tedious and physically demanding work, historian Rachel Maines (1999) argued that Dr J Mortimer Granville pioneered the labour-saving "vibrator" in the 1880s to induce these orgasms (though he himself denied its use for this purpose).

CHAPTER 3

A HISTORY OF SAME-SEX SEX

(by James)

Being a gay-identifying man in modern times, nothing really surprises me anymore. So I was delighted to be very surprised at how well documented the accepted practice of same-sex relations (at least amongst men) was in ancient times. Same-sex sex was seen as a normal rite of passage, pederasty (sex with adolescents) was commonplace, and there are many records documenting romantic love between same-sex couples. Ancient times were so much more "progressive" in these ways that, if it weren't for the Christian Church, early psychiatry and more recently the AIDS epidemic, modern-day same-sex sexpectations might have been very different.

PEDERASTY AND RITE OF PASSAGE

Mythology and stories of same-sex relations as a form of initiation to manhood can be traced back to Indo-European warriors. In the Germanic Tafali tribe, young men were paired with adult warriors and for the duration of their warrior training, would learn under them and have sex with them until the young men became adults and completed an initiation task such as killing a bear (Ammianus Marcellinus, fourth-century Roman writer). It can be deduced, therefore, that from the earliest recordings, same-sex sex was not only permissible, but was also seen as the path to "manhood".

Similarly, there is a record of the Cretans in the tribal pre-history of Greece engaging in ritual kidnapping. A boy from an elite background was taken by an aristocratic adult male, with the consent of the boy's father. The man took the boy out into the wilderness where they spent two months hunting, feasting and learning life skills, respect and responsibility. It is generally assumed that the man would begin having sex with the boy soon after taking him into the wilds. If the boy was pleased with how this went, he changed his status to comrade *(parastates),* signifying that he had fought in battle beside his mentor. He then returned to society and lived with him (Chrystal, 2016).

After the rise of the city-state in ancient Greece, boys would no longer go out into the wild, but rather pair up with older men and stay within the city for their education and instruction. This practice of pederasty occurred with boys from the age of approximately twelve until they grew body hair and became an adult at approximately seventeen years (Nussbaum, 1999).

To love a boy below the age of twelve years old was considered inappropriate but there is no evidence of any legal penalties attached to it. There is also a suggestion that the boys had some power and choice in these relationships, differentiating this practice from our modern definition of paedophilia; these boys were courted and showered with gifts and would withhold sex until they could determine if the mentor's intentions were honourable. Literature also suggests the boys would compete to attain the most desirable male partner by looking their best and frequenting the *gymnasia* (some things don't change, do they?). They could also denounce the mentor if he misbehaved in any way (Chrystal, 2016).

Perhaps this coming-of-age practice can be understood more fully if we consider that this ancient society believed the male sex drive to be an imperative and a possible threat to female chastity if left unsatisfied. For example, in the Azande tribe of north-west Africa, warriors achieved favourable status as "best" and "most trustworthy" when they owned a "wife-boy" (a young male sex slave) because they were seen as no threat towards women as a result (Barry, 1986).

A DIFFERENT WAY OF THINKING ABOUT SEXUALITY

Most people think of gender non-conformity – where a person's behaviour or gender expression does not match masculine or feminine gender norms – as a relatively new phenomenon. However, many ancient and traditional cultures embraced a wide range of sexualities, gender identities and gender expressions. Some Native American groups, for example, had a third and fourth gender category whereby people could live as the gender opposite to the one they were ascribed to at birth whilst still adhering to the more traditional gender roles. These "two-spirit" people were regarded as important and given special ceremonial roles (Roscoe, 1998).

In early Europe (i.e. ancient Greece and Rome), they had a different way of thinking about gender and sexuality as well. Rather than defining sexual preference as gender-based, they defined it by the role each participant played in the sex act. The active penetrator role was associated with masculinity, higher social status and adulthood. The passive penetrated role was seen as more feminine, low status and the role of youth (Halperin, 2012). Therefore, when intercourse occurred between two men it wasn't regarded as a homosexual union given that one partner would take on the passive role and therefore would no longer be considered a "man" in terms of the sexual union (Davidson, 2001). However, men who sold sex would always be the passive partner and receive (anally or "interfemorally" (between the thighs)) and were stripped of their civil rights because of this role.

Similarly, although same-sex sex was common amongst Nordic warriors, there was great stigma attached to being "*argr*", a term used to describe one who was feminine or acted "as a woman". It's said that these men would be humiliated and subjected to rape (Dynes, 1992). So it seems it was femininity and "bottoming" that was subject to prejudice, not same-sex sex per se, perhaps foreshadowing the contempt some modern-day (McGill, 2014) "bottoms" experience in the homosexual community.

Jacques Derrida (1968) called the phenomenon of basing our understanding of the human condition on the experiences of men "phallogocentrism", and we can see that from ancient Greek times that humans have prioritised the experience of penetration of the male penis. Historian Leila Rupp notes that whilst evidence of sex between women is present throughout history, they were framed by a male-centric conception of sex: "What we find historically and cross-culturally is … that sex was so defined by the participation of a penis that what women might do with their bodies did not count as sex" (Rupp, 2012).

As such, the historical record of love and sexual relations between women is sparse and the information we do have about early lesbianism is muddy. Plato's *Symposium* (191e) mentions women who "do not care for men, but have female attachments". The poet Sappho wrote about the beauty of women and her love of girls in the sixth century BC (Aldrich, 2006) but it is not known if these relationships were sexual. There are also vases depicting eroticised women: bathing, touching one another with dildos placed around the scene, but whether this eroticism is for the viewer (like ancient porn) or an accurate representation of same-sex sexuality is unknown (Bremmer, 1984).

Even during the Renaissance (1600s), lesbian relationships were regarded as harmless and incomparable to heterosexual ones unless the participants attempted to assert privileges and penetration traditionally enjoyed by men. We see during these times that hermaphroditism became synonymous with female same-sex desire, where women with longer, engorged clitorises were thought to penetrate other women – penetration once again being the focus of concern (Jennings, 2007).

Throughout the US, Europe and especially in England in the seventeenth to nineteenth centuries, women were accepted and even encouraged to express a passionate love for each other and there are many surviving love letters to document this. These "romantic friendships" were considered unthreatening and promoted as practice for a woman's marriage to a man (Faderman, 1981). Whether the relationship included any genital component was not mentioned, but women could form strong and exclusive bonds with each other and still be considered virtuous, innocent and chaste, whereas a similar relationship with a man would have ruined a woman's reputation.

SAME-SEX LOVE AND MARRIAGE

In ancient times, most of the adult men who engaged in same-sex sex would have been married (but not to each other). Marriage was seen as a duty and not a romantic engagement. Choosing to identify as homosexual or build a life with another man does not seem to have been a choice for men in most historical records. A notable exception being recorded in the community of the Siwa Oasis in south-west Egypt, where it is understood that a form of marriage between men was a regular practice (Fakhry, 1973).

However, there are records of romantic love between men. My favourite ancient love tale is that of Roman Emperor Hadrian and his mentee/lover Antinous (Lambert, Royston, 1984). Hadrian was Roman emperor from 117 AD to 138 AD. He was fond of arts and culture and, unlike the emperors before him, was not huge on military exercises. Hadrian was also fond of travel, and it was during a trip to Greece in 123 AD where he met a young boy by the name of Antinous.

Antinous was fit, smart and willing to learn – all features Hadrian apparently found attractive. As a result, Hadrian (who was forty-eight years old) took on Antinous (thirteen years old) as a mentee, having the young Greek follow him around on his travels and becoming part of Hadrian's retinue.

Alas like all classic love tales, this one too ended in tragedy when, on a trip down the Nile in 130 AD, Antinous drowned in strange circumstances. No one could conclude whether he was pushed, jumped himself or fell (though historians say that it most probably was an accident). However, what we can conclude is the very real romantic attachment of the Emperor to the boy.

Whilst still in Egypt, Hadrian had the local priesthood deify Antinous, glorifying him to a "divine level". He also had Antinous properly embalmed and mummified, and named a city after him. It is said that Hadrian howled with crying for what seemed like months and ordered the creation of approximately two thousand statues of Antinous after his death. How's that for dedication to your lover?

Another famous same-sex love tale occurred in the late 1500s, early 1600s between King James VI and I (he was king of Scotland and later became the king of England and Wales as well) and George Villiers, who eventually became the Duke of Buckingham. It is said that the two men were notorious for kissing and caressing each other in public, and that their heedless contempt for public opinion contributed to the civil crisis that was enveloping the nation (Norton, 1998).

Just as Emperor Hadrian was married, King James VI and I also had a wife and three children. So although it's safe to say that whilst we have records of powerful love between men, these men were still expected to follow heterosexual convention in their family lives. Similarly, Queen Christina of Sweden chose to abdicate the throne in 1654 to avoid heterosexual marriage, we assume due to her preference to dress as a man and pursue relationships with women (Faderman, 1981).

HOMOSEXUALITY, RELIGION AND LAW

Although there are a lot of references to same-sex relationships in the Bible, the historical Christian Church was generally anti-homosexuality and had, at times, used its great influence to influence law-making in this regard (Shorter, 2005; Tannahill, 2006). The Renaissance saw intense oppression of same-sex sex by the Roman Catholic Church and during this time same-sex sex went from being completely legal to incurring the death penalty in most parts of Europe (Boswell, 1980).

The Holy Roman Empire made sodomy punishable by death in 1532 (Fone, 2000). Following suit, Henry VIII criminalised sodomy in England in 1533. The new statue outlawed the "detestable and abominable vice of buggery committed with mankind or beast". The offence was punishable by death, and could be tried in the secular court.

At a similar time in France, first-offending "sodomites" lost their testicles, second offenders lost their penis, and third offenders were burned. Women caught in same-sex acts would be mutilated and executed as well.

Between 1540 and 1700, over 1,600 people were prosecuted for sodomy (Fone, 2000). Buggery remained a capital offence in England until 1861, after which it was downgraded but still a punishable offence.

Although same-sex sexual acts were decriminalised in several countries before 1900 (including France, Belgium, the Netherlands, Argentina, Brazil and Mexico), they remained criminal in Britain and all of its colonies until the twentieth century. Many might be surprised to learn that many states in the United States only decriminalised sodomy in 2003!

In fact, British colonisation took institutionalised homophobia to countries that never before had issues with same-sex relations, such as China, Japan, India and parts of Africa.

To this day, there are still seventy United Nations member states that criminalise same-sex sexual acts. Six of those penalise it with the death penalty (R.L. Mendos, 2019).

PSYCHIATRY AND SAME-SEX SEX

Because same-sex sex was considered "unnatural" until the nineteenth century, people became interested in discovering the cause of same-sex attraction, presumably to eradicate it. Therefore, medicine and psychiatry took over from law and religion as the authority on the "disorder" and these disciplines began to study homosexuality scientifically.

At this time, most theories regarded homosexuality as a disease, but in the mid-twentieth century there was a paradigm shift and psychiatrists began to believe same-sex attraction could be cured through therapy. Some early psychiatrists such as Sigmund Freud and Havelock Ellis adopted tolerant stances on homosexuality. Freud and Ellis believed that homosexuality was not normal, but for some people was "unavoidable".

Alfred Kinsey's research and publications (1948 and 1953), however, found great variability of sexual preference on a scale from exclusively homosexual to exclusively heterosexual. This work began the large-scale social and cultural shift away from the view that homosexuality was an abnormal condition. Kinsey's books demonstrated that same-sex sex was more common than was assumed, suggesting that these behaviours were normal and part of a continuum of sexual behaviours.

As such, even though homosexuality was placed as a disorder in the first version of the *Diagnostic Statistical Manual* in 1952, in 1973 it was edited to only include ego-dystonic homosexuality (when you feel same-sex desire but don't identify as homosexual), before being removed in its entirety in 1987.

HIV AND AIDS

The late 70's to early 80's marked the decriminalisation of homosexuality throughout much of the developed world. For the first time, gay men and lesbians could express their love publicly without fear of a criminal conviction, so the parties began. The euphoria of this sexual nirvana was short lived as a dark cloud in the form of a "gay cancer" began killing young, fit gay men in the prime of their lives.

Gay and bisexual men in New York, San Francisco and Los Angeles were unexpectedly falling ill with flu-like symptoms, rare cancers and skin diseases that had only ever been found in developing countries. Within six months, many died. By the mid 80s the virus causing these deaths had been named HIV and its reach had gone global. From the UK to Australia, from South America to South Africa, the virus sent shock-waves throughout gay communities.

WHAT IS HIV?

Human Immunodeficiency Virus (HIV) is a blood-borne virus that is primarily transmitted via contact of blood, semen, breast milk, pre-ejaculate and vaginal fluids. Essentially, the virus kills off blood cells (CD4+ T cells) that help protect the body from acquiring infections. If left untreated, HIV can turn into AIDS (Acquired Immunodeficiency Syndrome), disabling the body's immune system, allowing infections, viruses, diseases and cancers to thrive, slowly shutting down organs and leading ultimately to death.

There are fewer cases of AIDS in the developed world today thanks to advances in medication. However, in developing nations throughout South Africa, the Pacific Islands, South America, Asia and Russia, HIV and AIDS remain a major public health issue.

Politics, access to testing and treatment, stigma and cultural barriers continue to perpetuate HIV, particularly in the poorest regions of the globe. Whilst someone diagnosed HIV positive in Australia today can expect to lead a full and productive life, stigma and pollical willpower remain the greatest obstacles in the eradication of the virus.

To say the infection had a devastating effect on the gay community would be a gross understatement. For years, friends of gay men were going to funeral after funeral wondering who would be next. Gay clubs that used to be throbbing with activity in dark backrooms soon had a ghost-like feeling about them, with men terrified they might catch the then-deadly virus. Thus, male same-sex sex grew to carry a great stigma, gay men were called diseased and people worried that kissing or even touching an infected person might transfer the virus.

Whilst the virus spread, condoms were promoted as the only way to keep yourself protected from infection (apart from refraining from sex altogether). At the same time, porn production houses started fetishising men having "bareback" sex, and men reported that condoms made them feel disconnected during sex, which ironically elevated the desirability of unprotected sex (Mowlabocus et al., 2013).

The government health campaigns aimed at stopping the spread of HIV often did more to stigmatise the disease and people living with it than help to prevent infection. For example, in Australia, the campaign depicted the virus as a Grim Reaper, knocking down women, children and men with bowling balls at a ten-pin bowling lane. As a counter-effort, a lot of work started to be done to research and raise awareness of the disease. In 1989, Madonna even famously included an information flyer titled 'The Facts About AIDS', aimed at de-stigmatising the virus and educating people, in every copy of her album *Like a Prayer*.

Continued destigmatisation has coincided with the advances in medical technology that allow people living with HIV to live regular, healthy lives with equal life expectancy to that of someone not living with HIV. There is now a lot of hope in the medical and HIV-advocacy community that we will one day see the end of this virus.

CHAPTER 4

SEXPECTATIONS AFTER THE SEXUAL REVOLUTION

The Sexual Revolution was the name given to the social movement grouping together a series of significant cultural events from the 1960s to the 1980s that challenged traditional sex and relationship norms. These events included the increased acceptance of pre-marital sex, the legalisation of abortion, and the normalisation of contraception, pornography, nudity, masturbation and homosexuality. Thus, the "second" Sexual Revolution (the official first revolution was in the 1920s) can be credited for inspiring many of the sexpectations we have today.

THE PILL

Condoms made from materials such as fish bladders, linen sheaths and animal intestines have been around since approximately 3000 BC. The ancient Egyptians would mix a paste out of crocodile dung and form it into a pessary to be inserted into the vagina to prevent pregnancy. Aristotle proposed cedar oil and frankincense oil as spermicides and Casanova wrote of using half a lemon as a cervical cap (Lipsey et al., 2005). Despite these diverse forms of contraception invented and used throughout the ages, many people argue that the oral contraceptive pill (aka "the Pill") was largely responsible for the Sexual Revolution (Liao & Dollin, 2012).

Sixty years after its invention, we take the Pill for granted, yet it holds a unique place in contraceptive history. It is credited as being the first form of contraception that was wholly controlled by women, easy to use and inexpensive, a genuine and therefore "respectable" medical product, relatively safe, highly effective and taken separate from the sexual act – separating the act of sex from the function of procreation (Liao & Dollin, 2012).

Some people have argued that the Pill was merely released at the right time, coinciding with the liberalisation of attitudes rather than causing them (May, 2010). However, there is no doubt about its popularity – the number of women taking it climbed from roughly four hundred thousand in 1961 to 1.2 million a year later, then triple that in 1965 (Gibbs, 2010). Personal reports also reveal the Pill as having a profound emotional impact on women's experience of their sexuality.

'I was too scared of getting pregnant to risk using nothing, though my boyfriend tried to convince me. So, I got a diaphragm from my doctor – and hated it … but the second I went on the Pill, all the mess and the worry and holding my breath every month to see if I got my period was completely lifted off my shoulders.' – **Mary**

The Pill was approved by the American FDA in 1960 and was legalised for married couples in the United States in

1965, and for unmarried women in 1972. By 1971, more than 75% of Americans thought that premarital sex was acceptable, a threefold increase from the 1950s. Because women could have sex before marriage without risk of getting pregnant, they could also delay marriage and/or having children in order to pursue education and careers. As such, the number of unmarried Americans aged twenty to twenty-four more than doubled from 1960 to 1976 (Villaverde et al., 2014).

Interestingly, although the Pill emancipated women from the roles of wife and mother, early feminists such as Germaine Greer criticised the Pill as benefiting men more than women because it removed an acceptable reason for refusing sex. "Once they had made the investment in sexual activity by taking a daily medication in order to be available, there was no sense in being unavailable. Having accepted the idea of themselves as sexually active, they had to be sexually active or be failures" (Greer quoted in Cooke, 2010).

PORNOGRAPHY

Forms of explicit imagery have been around since prehistoric times. However, modern pornography – roughly defined as material designed solely for sexual arousal, without artistic merit – can be seen to have been legitimised with Hugh Hefner's *Playboy* magazine in 1953 (Schuchardt, 2003). Following the success of *Playboy*, bans on books with explicit erotic content (such as the 1740 John Cleland novel *Fanny Hill*, widely known to be the first English pornographic novel) were challenged and overturned both in the United States and in the UK during the period of 1959 to 1966. This paved the way for the 1973 US Supreme Court decision to narrow the definition of obscenity, resulting in fewer prosecutions for pornography.

As for film, Denmark was the first country to decriminalise pornography by removing censorship laws in 1969. This year marked the beginning of what is now known as the Golden Age of Pornography when many erotic films received mainstream attention and the porn industry was born on a mass scale. The first of these was Andy Warhol's *Blue Movie* (1969), which shows a heterosexual couple having sex.

When the videocassette recorders (VCRs) entered homes in the 1980s more than 75% of the tapes sold were porn. So much was the power of porn that it became widely accepted that global electronics company Sony's decision to ban porn from its competing Betamax doomed it to oblivion (Kushner, 2019). VCRs made it possible for people to watch movies at home instead of at sketchy adult theatres on the wrong side of town; porn was suddenly a lot more accessible.

However, the most important development in the history of pornography was the internet and the anonymity and privacy it brought. By turning on your computer (and in the 1990s, dialling up) porn was suddenly easily, privately and freely accessible. When porn shifted from publicly purchased VCRs and publicly viewed films to privately viewed internet downloads, the type of sex shown on screen shifted too. From the safety and anonymity of their home, more men began to watch fetish porn, depicting specific, sometimes odd, sexual behaviour.

> *Thirty years ago "hard-core" pornography usually meant the explicit depiction of sexual intercourse … Now hard-core has evolved and is increasingly dominated by the sadomasochistic themes … all involving scripts fusing sex with hatred and humiliation. Hard-core pornography now explores the world of*

perversion, whilst soft-core is what hard-core was a few decades
ago … The comparatively tame soft-core pictures of yesteryear now
show up on mainstream media all day long, in the pornification
of everything, including television, rock videos, soap operas,
advertisements, and so on.' (Doige, 2007)

No one keeps official records so the actual size of the porn
industry today is a mystery. We can, however, assume that it
is a multi-billion dollar business with conservative estimates
that the internet is made up of 4–14% pornography (Ward,
2013). Regardless of how big the online porn industry is, we
know it is being viewed. Most studies put porn use in the last
week at about 80% for men and 30% for women.

With porn use being so prevalent, it's little wonder that it
has a major influence on our sexpectations. The effects of
pornography exposure upon older adolescents and young
adults were comprehensively studied as early as the 1980s in
a research series conducted by Dolf Zillmann and Jennings
Bryant (Zillmann & Bryant, 1988; Manning, 2006). These
studies found that even before the proliferation of porn on
the internet, viewing porn over only six weeks had a raft of
effects. The studies were so conclusive and effects seen as so
detrimental that they could not get the ethics approval to re-
run them (Paul, 2010)! The effects included:

- Men demonstrated increased callousness towards women.
- Subjects considered the crime of rape less serious and
  reported increased acceptance of male dominance and
  female servitude.
- Subjects were more accepting of non-marital sexual activity,
  sexual infidelity, and non-coital sexual practices such as oral
  and anal sex.

- Subjects became more interested in more extreme and deviant forms of pornography.
- Subjects were more likely to say they were dissatisfied with their sexual partner.
- Subjects valued marriage less and were twice as likely to believe marriage may become obsolete. They reported greater tolerance of non-exclusive sexual access to intimate partners.
- Men experienced a decreased desire to become fathers, and women experienced a decreased desire to have a daughter.
- Subjects showed a greater acceptance of male and female promiscuity and the belief that the repression of sexual inclinations poses a health risk.

Porn can also give a distorted view of the role of sex in relationships, including an overestimation of how much sex people are having, normalisation of sexual promiscuity, and negative beliefs around sexual abstinence. There is strong evidence that exposure to violent pornography is associated with sexually aggressive behaviours in men (Ybarra et al., 2011.; Hald, et al., 2010). Additionally, women who have viewed pornography report increased participation in anal sex despite data that the majority of women consider anal sex unpleasant (Tryden et al., 2001).

... And that is if porn doesn't replace sex entirely for some people! One recent study showed 20% of men who are regular pornography users preferred the excitement of viewing pornography over being sexually intimate with a real person (Sznitter, 2012).

PORN DISCOVERY AND SAME-SEX-ATTRACTED PEOPLE
(By James)

Gay and bisexual men have a slightly different relationship with porn than our heterosexual counterparts. Whilst hetero sex and relationships were all around us, in TV shows, movies, magazines and everywhere in our real lives, gay kids growing up before the new millennium had to look to porn to find any examples of two guys fucking.

Sex education in schools has been mediocre at best for heterosexuals, but the near exclusion of any same-sex sex education in schools has meant that a whole generation of young same-sex attracted people have had to get their sex education from porn. Even today, only heterosexual sex is included in the formal curriculum in schools (Pascoe, 2012). Indeed, research has found that searching for sexual health information online varies significantly by sexual orientation. In one study, only 19% of heterosexual youths compared to 78% of gay/lesbian/queer youths looked for information about sex online. They reported that they did this because they didn't have anyone to ask (Mitchell et al., 2014).

I remember doing internet searches on "hot men" and "men having sex" and "sperm" (I know, not very creative) when I was a teenager, just to see what happened or if men even had sex with each other. Growing up in rural Australia, there weren't any gay people around that I was aware of, and the only evidence I had that gays existed was from the movie *Priscilla: Queen of the Desert* – I was hoping I'd find something on the internet that didn't involve me having to get frocked up!

Unfortunately, I made a rookie error and forgot to clear the search history on our family computer. My parents stumbled across what I'd been looking for, which led to a very embarrassing conversation where I tried to convince them that I was "just seeing what gay people did". I'm certain that my parents didn't believe me for a moment. I was much more careful to delete all my internet history after that.

Porn can have negative effects on the sexpectations of gay and bi men as well. There's the unrealistic dick sizes, the expectations around how far or how much you can blow, how long sex lasts, how much force is used when having sex, and what you think is enjoyable. Some may argue that porn is also responsible for fetishising traditionally risky gay sex acts such as bareback sex, the intentional spread of HIV (chasing) and chemsex. However, academics argue there is a big difference between fantasising about an act or activity, and actually following through with it (Rosewarne, 2011).

It would be amiss to say all porn is bad for same-sex sex education. Early same-sex porn had the ability to teach same-sex attracted people about condom use, the logistics of the act, and helped them explore different fetishes. Most importantly, porn allowed young people to realise they were not alone in their sexual attraction or desires.

Today, we have many more ways young or curious same-sex attracted people can learn about same-sex relationships. Now many plotlines in popular culture actually celebrate LGBT+ relationships, normalising them, rather than storylines where we get killed or assaulted. We also have songs, singers, plays, radio programmes – you name it. Not to mention LGBT+ organisations publishing their own sex and relationships advice and guidelines to help those who want more information. And we still have porn.

Porn can be a force for good, but only by increasing awareness about how porn is made, why it's made and how we can manage our expectations to not be damaged by porn will we all be better off.

FREE LOVE, DIVORCE AND DIFFERENT RELATIONSHIP MODELS

The mid-1960s marked a move away from the traditional relationship model of monogamous, heterosexual, "till-death-do-us-part" marriage. A new culture of "free love" emerged inspired by Indian culture. The "hippies" that are now synonymous with the free-love movement expressed contempt for the cultural norms of the 1950s and encouraged spiritual question, sexual liberation and experimentation with drugs. The hippie movement achieved its height during the summer of 1967 (known as "The Summer of Love") when as many as one hundred thousand people converged in San Francisco's neighbourhood of Haight-Ashbury.

At the same time, the gay rights movement began and has since been symbolised by the Stonewall riots of 1969. The riots were a series of spontaneous violent demonstrations by members of the LGBT+ community against a police raid of the Stonewall Inn in New York City. The riots increased public awareness of gay rights and allowed many gay men to "come out" and live full time as a homosexual, no longer living in secret and having to sneak around.

As a result of the emergence of more liberal attitudes, sexual experimentation started to occur earlier in life, pushing marriage back to later in life. Women were encouraged to participate in and enjoy sex and move away from "the housewife" model of femininity by books such as *The Feminine Mystique* (Friedan, 1963). Swingers clubs were organised, first in suburban homes and later in public venues. One of the most well known of these was opened in 1977 in New York called Plato's Retreat.

The main goal of marriage following the Sexual Revolution became personal happiness and self-fulfilment (Bellah et al.,1985; Cherlin, 2004; Popenoe, 1996). People's sexpectations of pleasure and sexual satisfaction within marriage also increased (Seidman, 1991). However, because marriages held together by mutual satisfaction are intrinsically less stable than are marriages held together by community expectations, legal requirements, and religious restrictions, the long-term rise in divorce became inevitable. Spouses tended to seek divorces when they became dissatisfied with their relationships, no longer willing to remain married through the difficult times (Popenoe, 1996).

The "no-fault" unilateral divorce became legal and easier to obtain in many countries between the 1960s and 1980s. Under the new legislation, the first of which was passed in California in 1969, only one ground for divorce existed: that the marriage was "irretrievably broken" as a result of "irreconcilable differences" (Glendon, 1989). Moreover, courts granted divorces even if one spouse wanted the divorce and the other did not (hence the "unilateral"). This made divorce easier and by the end of the 1970s, the great majority of Americans viewed divorce as an unfortunate but common event, and thus the stigma of divorce reduced.

More than forty years after these social and cultural changes, the ideals of the Sexual Revolution have become implicit and unquestioned in our society. We are free and open with our sexuality, and there is far more acceptance for various sexual preferences and relationship models. However, sexual liberation has begun to face its own challenges in the rise of the #MeToo movement. Growing reports of women being pressured to exchange sexual favours for career advancement has led to the discussion of "consent" in earnest. Neither Hollywood movies nor pornography (especially porn!) portray couples talking to each other and asking questions before or during sex. Sex is presented as a passionate, erotic and always enjoyable encounter born out of the "heat of the moment". With no cultural modelling to draw from, progressive authors are now openly discussing the need for more conversation and education on what constitutes "explicit and enthusiastic" consent.

PART 1: SUMMARY & EXERCISES

Our sexpectations determine our satisfaction with our sex lives, and each of our personal sexpectations are influenced by a multitude of factors. Not only are we influenced by our own culture and era, we inherit the sexpectations of previous generations and times in history passed down through dogma and taboo. No matter where you identify on the sexual spectrum, you can guarantee that you have been influenced not only by your family, friends and media exposure but also by generations of people and eras before you.

So, to encourage your understanding of the history behind your own sexpectations, have a go at answering the following questions.

1   From the history you have just read, was there anything that may have been passed down to you? Did you recognise any of the sexpectations in your own beliefs or attitudes about sex?
2   Thinking about your own culture and era, what is the role and function of sex in your society? How are people in your culture *supposed* to be, sexually speaking?
3   How did you come to know these sexpectations?
4   If you could write your own sexual rulebook, at this point what would be your "prescriptions" (what I should do) and

"prohibitions" (what I shouldn't do)? What "permissions" would be useful to have?

See below for some examples:

Prescriptions:

- I should practise safe sex.
- I should have sex with multiple people before "settling down".
- I should orgasm and ensure my partner orgasms.
- I should experience desire and "chemistry" with my sexual partner.

Prohibitions:

- I should not fake an orgasm.
- I should not say no to sex too often.
- I should not be interested in anyone else when I'm in love with a partner.
- I should not be too "easy".

Permissions:

- It's okay to want sex sometimes and not at other times, or not want it at all.
- It's okay to have sex for reasons other than lust or desire and with people you don't have "chemistry" with.
- It's okay to not be interested in sexual experimentation.
- It's okay to be selfish in bed.
- It's okay for not all sex to lead to intercourse.

PART 2

SEXPECTATIONS TODAY

[We are all having the sex we *think* we want]

CHAPTER 5

YOUR SEXPECTATIONS

FINDING YOUR TRUTH

Compared to past eras, it could be said that we have relative sexual freedom and a plethora of information about sex to inform and develop our own sexpectations. Film and internet technology have made the dissemination of information easy. Contraception and the Sexual Revolution have lifted some of the stigma on female and same-sex sexuality. Therefore, even though our sex education in schools is arguably still somewhat lacking, we often reach adulthood with at least some understanding of sex.

Not only do we have more knowledge than previous generations, but our current cultural sexpectations are much greater. We expect a lot from our sex lives, our sexual partners, and from our bodies. The pressures we place around sex are so great that recent surveys in the US and UK report that approximately one in three women believe they are not as interested in sex as they should be and one in four men believe they don't last as long as they think they should. It is safe to say that we are no more frigid or dysfunctional than in previous times, it's just that the sexpectations we have internalised are working to make many of us more insecure!

There are sexpectations all around us, whether we realise it or not. When you chat with friends, pick up a magazine, in your religious service, on the news, at the doctor's surgery, on the TV, at the movies, on billboards and in advertising, in social media, porn and on dating apps. Because these messages are similar and ubiquitous, they often feel "normal" or "natural" rather than just one possible way of thinking about sex. We end up absorbing them unconsciously, acting on them and sharing the same ideas when we ourselves talk about sex.

However, culture isn't the only thing that determines our sexpectations. Simon and Gagnon's (1999) sexual script theory also identifies the importance of the interpersonal and intrapsychic levels on which we form sexual scripts (another term for sexpectations). They propose that cultural ideas of sexual behaviour are collectively developed and communicated through social institutions (e.g. schools, TV), then the individual develops their own sexual scripts, identity and practices at the interpersonal level – with friends, social groups and partners (Gagnon, 1973). Finally, we can also form intrapsychic scripts – meaning we can develop a sex life in our head through our fantasies that we may or may not act upon. As such, we can define our sexual preferences and sexpectations similarly or differently to those we find in our culture or relationships, and enact them interpersonally or keep them private.

If we choose to define our sexual selves differently to social norms, we may experience pressure to conform. Social pressure can take many forms including direct criticism, marginalisation, bullying and ostracism.

'I wanted to wait until it would be special but I didn't want to be called frigid and be left out. In the end, I lost it with some guy I met at a party, in his car. It wasn't great but at least people got off my case from then on.' – **Tracey**

Bowing to social pressure can occur in three main ways: compliance, identification and internalisation. If you comply, you will go along with what is believed to be "normal" in public but your private beliefs remain unchanged.

'I remember being a teenager and hearing the guys talk about pussy. I knew I was different and I wasn't into girls, but I went along with it anyway, you know, just to fit in.' – **Jake**

If you experience identification, your public behaviour and private beliefs are changed, but only whilst you are in the presence of your social group.

'When I was in the community, kink was everything to me. I lived and breathed it and felt it was such an important part of who I was, what made me special and sexy … since meeting my partner I rarely go to [kink] events and I don't miss it. Turns out it was a phase or something …' – **Heidi**

With internalisation, the deepest level of conformity, both your public behaviour and private beliefs are changed again but this time unconsciously. In psychology we call this adoption of other's beliefs and values as if it were your own truth "introjection" (Rogers, 1951). Rogers believed that introjected values or beliefs can get in the way of people being their true selves. Because these values become so deeply ingrained out of our conscious awareness, it feels like "truth" and is perceived as therefore immutable regardless of whether these beliefs are helping or hindering you.

Just as you can't consent to sex when you are unconscious, you can't have any meaningful choice when the sexpectations – the sexual dogma that influence you – are unconscious. To adopt a sexpectation as your own authentic preference, you have to be aware that these are, indeed, sexpectations and not immutable truths. When we aren't aware, we base our sex lives on these sexpectations rather than listening to what our bodies are telling us we *really* want.

Differentiating "truth" from "dogma" is a very tricky task in current times when the scientific model reigns supreme and certain data is presented as medical "facts". However, just as in medieval times medicine "knew" that the seminal humour needed to be balanced and in the 1800s it was medical "fact" that the female orgasm affected fertility, what is described as science in the current discourse around sexuality could in fact be seen as dogma in years to come. I mean we still don't "know" the origins of same-sex attraction … Are we really all that much more advanced than our medieval predecessors?

WHAT ARE YOUR SEXPECTATIONS OF "GOOD SEX"?

So what sexpectations are you influenced by? In posing the below questions, I want to acknowledge the training I received from Dr Sandra Pertot – a sex educator who first made me aware of my own unconscious beliefs around sex and thus began my thinking around the concept of sexpectations. These questions, adapted from those Dr Pertot posed to us, will help you assess what you take for granted about sex and relationships. It may be a starting point for you to see which sexpectations may be causing problems in your sex life and relationships, stopping you from having the sex that will really fulfil you.

If you are in a sexual relationship, it can also be useful to compare your responses with your partner's. If you don't currently have a regular sexual partner, it can be useful to think back to past partners and experiences to deduce what that person's sexpectations may have been that caused them to be sexual with you in their specific way.

1. MEMORIES:

Think back to the best (or one of the best) sexual experience/s you have had. Describe it in as much detail as you can remember.

Based on this memory, what can you see are the defining qualities of great sex for you?

For example:

One of my best sexual experiences was on our summer holidays. We had nothing to do and nothing on our minds except each other. The day was spent lazily and in the nude. We would have slow sex, hot sex, against-the-wall sex, in-the-shower sex, interspersed with little intimacies – a game of cards, reading the paper out loud, making sandwiches. There was no agenda, no timeframe. We knew each other's bodies and turn-ons the way long-time lovers do. Lazing in the afterglow on top of the bed covers, our bodies slick and slippery, with the cool air from the overhead fan dancing over us. I have no idea how many times we had sex but my body stayed in a constant state of turn-on all day. Reading books whilst spooning on the couch, my fingers would draw patterns on his skin, our hands magnetically drawn to each other. Making tea in the kitchen, I'd look over and watch him moving about unselfconsciously, watching the light play over the hard planes of his body, and I'd just want to jump him all over again.

The above example illustrates that great sex for me can be about intimacy and comfort with a partner. It's about the freedom to take time, to be with a partner with no distractions. It's just as much about the intimacy that happens outside of sex as during it.

It is interesting that this is the memory that came up for me. I have had many experiences of what I consider "great sex" and many of these are quite different in both content and qualities to what I described above. However, I haven't been in a long-term intimate relationship for many years. I imagine these current circumstances influence my fond memory for the small intimacies of long-term lovers.

With this in mind, perhaps you might compare the qualities in the first memory that came to your mind with another two to see if your themes of "great sex" are consistent or varied. Do you have any insight as to why the qualities you have identified might be important to you now?

2. VALUES:

As you read this list of values, identify those that reflect what you think are important in your sex life. Don't pick the ones that just sound attractive; pick the ones that you think influence how you think, act and help create your experience of your sex life. It's not a complete list, so feel free to add any that better reflect your experience.

Begin by circling the ten most important values to you, then narrow down your preference to your top three. Which three values are the least important to you?

Risk
Delight
Presence
Sensuality
Expertise
Respect
Connection
Intimacy
Gentleness
Love
Understanding
Stimulation
Attractiveness
Empathy
Relaxation
Tenderness
Laughter
Satisfaction: partner
Consideration
Frequent
Satisfaction: self
Honesty
Responsiveness
Fun
Spirituality
Acceptance

Experimentation
Bliss
Play
Giving
Performance
Encouragement
Power
Control
Passion
Trust
Excitement
Novelty
Spontaneity
Friendship
Mystery
Vigour
Submission
Dominance
Desire
Challenge
Growth
Pleasure
Exhibition
Status
Validation

You might begin to see some themes emerging for you in the last two exercises. Perhaps some of the qualities you were able to draw out of your "great sex" memory are similar to the values you identified. For example, I relate to the values of *sensuality* and *presence* and you can pick this out in my great sex story through the sensuality in my description (e.g. the memory of the cooling breeze of the fan) and the sense of presence implied through being able to focus totally on each other.

You may also start to discover where some sexual experiences or connections have been "off" for you. One couple I used to see for sex therapy had been living together for two years and complained of loss of desire and sex in their relationship. When we looked at their sexual values, one of them picked out *intimacy*, *tenderness* and *connection*. The other picked out *novelty*, *passion* and *spontaneity*. You can see from their very different ideas on what was important in sex where they might have experienced a sexual disconnection! Luckily, helping them understand how they were different also helped them to give each other what each of them really wanted.

JAMES SAYS:

It might be difficult for you to narrow down this list to just three top qualities. It might depend on how you're feeling at the time or where you're at in your life. For me, there have been times where I related to a range of these values that are very different to what I currently feel. But if I think about the best (memorable!) sex I've had, funnily enough, I come up with the same values as Gemma – sensuality and presence. I'm also going to add in passion.

I've had a lot of sex in my time, and Lord knows there are a lot of experiences I don't remember. They might have been good experiences, but nothing stood out for me that would warrant it being memorable – I have been known to go on a date with someone for a second time, years later, without realising until thirty minutes in!

But if I think about a sexual experience that I will never forget because of how great it was, I don't have to look very hard. There were days, if not weeks, of mental foreplay. Talking back and forth with cute and sexy messages. Then, when we were finally together, it was passionate with no inhibitions and no worries about the time or the situation we were in. We were free to enjoy each other's company in that moment without thinking about anything else. There was clear communication, not just to let each other know how we were feeling throughout the night, but also allowing us to be in tune with our bodies. There was also no pressure on penetration occurring. Sure, there was penetration in the end, but it was a spur-of-the-moment decision because we were enjoying what was going on.

At times, I value risk, fun, excitement and control, but when I really narrow it down, sensuality, presence and passion come out on top.

3. GOAL POSTS:

- How long does a good session last?
- How does it end?
- What makes a great lover?
- What is good sexual communication?
- In a long-term relationship how often would you ideally have sex?

Through my work as a sex therapist, it has amazed me at how similar the sexpectations are that my clients hold. The summary of standard heterosexual sexpectations below comes from what I have understood through conversations with clients in therapy, from internet forums and in personal communications with my long-suffering friends (#sexnerd!). Compare your answers to the questions above to these common stereotypes.

In general I find that most people I speak to hold sexpectations that great sex is varied, passionate and that it lasts thirty minutes or more. Most people would see it as involving more than missionary position and with both partners as enthusiastic active participants (even if one is more dominant or leading the experience). Most people think that for great sex, both partners need to have an orgasm and, when having sex with a man, an erection is essential. In heterosexual sex, simultaneous orgasm is generally the ideal but as long as the man orgasms after the woman it can still meet the standard. Usually the experience is declared as "over" once the male comes to orgasm.

A great lover is often seen as one who has a great body, can control their own bodily responses, knows how to please a partner and expresses their own pleasure freely. Interestingly, a great lover is thought not to need to ask about what their partner likes, but should just "know". Many people (particularly if they have not been exposed to kink) think that good sexual communication therefore is a series of groans and sexy sounds, and that there is something wrong if directions need to be given.

How often people want to have sex generally relates to their sex drive. People with a higher sex drive tend to have higher ideals when it comes to sexual frequency. In our culture, having a high sex drive is valued, and in couples sex therapy it is often the partner with the lower drive who is presented as needing to be "fixed" when this isn't always the case.

According to the Australian Study of Health and Relationships (Richters et al., 2014), most people in long-term (greater than twelve months) monogamous relationships (including both hetero and same-sex oriented) say they would like to have sex between two and four times per week. However, on average most people have sex 1.4 times per week, which has decreased from the survey done in 2003 when the average was 1.8 times. Similarly in the US, a study (Twenge, Sherman & Wells, 2017) found that cohabiting couples have sex about once per week (fifty-one times a year) and that this figure has dropped since the early 1990s (by nine times a year) – a finding they attributed to an increasing number of people without a steady sexual partner and a decline in sexual frequency amongst those with partners.

SAME-SEX GOAL POST
(By James)

There are many similarities between same-sex sex and heterosexual sex in terms of what often constitutes "good sex", but it really depends on the person and the role they're playing in the situation. Let's have a look at the stereotypes of same-sex sex that I have gleaned from the people I have spoken to in my research for the sex radio shows I worked on, as well as my personal conversations. These stereotypes can apply to all genders except for where otherwise indicated.

People who are "tops" or perform an active role are expected to also maintain an erection (if they have a penis!) and take control in most scenarios. Those who are "bottoms" or play a passive role are expected to have no issues with being penetrated and performing oral sex. This is, of course, unless we're in a "power bottom" situation, where the bottom is more active in the role. For instance, riding the top whilst the top essentially lies there. Those who are versatile might perform all roles during sex and "flip" to change positions and states.

Unlike sex with heterosexuals, same-sex sex is not always over after a man orgasms. With men, sex could continue until the other male cums, or they might finish the remaining partner off by jerking them off or another activity. If the partner being penetrated cums first, penetrative sex is usually over, but that's not always the case. With same-sex-oriented women, orgasm might be just the beginning of more sex and penetration (with a dildo, strap-on, etc.) may or may not feature in a great sexual encounter.

As for duration of sex, that's totally up to the person you're with, the scenario you're in and what you feel like. Unlike heterosexuals, there's usually a lot of verbal communication between partners about what is happening and what might happen next, whether something feels good, and if it doesn't.

As with heterosexuals, in same-sex culture high sex drive is also valued in men and women. Gay men especially are expected to not just have high sex drives, but have a lot of sex. Many gay men, in my experience, have no idea how many sexual partners they've had in their lives.

4. INITIATION:

- Who initiates?
- How do they initiate?
- Why do they initiate?
- When is it okay to say no?
- And how does the partner deal with this?
- Is routine sex a sign of a poor sex life?

Most people believe that in a heterosexual relationship either the male partner should initiate or that each partner should initiate equally. This relates to cultural beliefs about the male sex drive being higher and therefore men "needing" more sex. Initiation is once again idealised as being non-verbal touch on non-genital zones, such as the arms or thighs, that communicates sexual interest and which is received positively by a partner.

In most people's sexpectations, great sex is initiated out of desire and passion for a partner. Because of our current elevation of high sex drives, and the ideals of mutual desire and passion, saying no to sex with your partner in a relationship is not well accepted. Therefore, despite our current-day emphasis on sexual consent, most people have conflicting beliefs about sexual refusal.

We generally believe in and endorse anyone's right to say no, and acknowledge that for various reasons (tiredness, stress, pain, not in the mood, etc.) it's okay to not want sex. However, in practice we will experience emotions like guilt, anxiety and shame if we say no too often, "lead someone on" or act "frigid". Although issues of consent and the #MeToo movement have mainly focused on women's consent, those identifying as male often have an even harder time being okay with saying no to their partner (due to male gender stereotypes) than those identifying as women do.

With a similar conflict of belief against experience, most people believe that a partner should accept a no with patience and equanimity. However, because of our cultural elevation of high sex drive, we believe that people "should" want sex, and therefore take it more personally if we get rejected. What is wrong with us? Aren't we attractive? We deserve sex! Despite our ideals, in reality we often get blinded by these beliefs, and many people will experience disappointment, insecurity, sulking, bargaining, frustration or anger when a sexual overture is rejected.

Spontaneity is linked with passion in our sexual ideals. We have very few examples in movies or pornography where sex is not portrayed as lust-fuelled and spontaneous. Routine sex is therefore often seen as less than optimal as it suggests an absence of desire. Many couples who last past the "honeymoon period" (where New Relationship Energy (NRE) stimulates sexual desire) will report that scheduling time to have sex is an important part of maintaining regular sexual contact. However, in our sexpectations, treating sex like a household chore and scheduling it removes the lust and romance we like to associate with our sex lives.

'People are always horrified when you tell them that you have to schedule sex, because they want it to be spontaneous and to fall from the heavens whilst you're folding the laundry. But sex only happens if you make it happen.' (Perel, 2017)

The same can be said for same-sex relationships. The main aspect that differs though is initiation. When both partners identify as the same sex, who initiates? Although sex could be initiated by either person, usually initiation will come from the person with the higher sex drive, or who is more confident or dominant.

5. MEANING:

- Why would you be distressed if you didn't have "good" sex?
- What is the meaning of sexual problems?
- What are the consequences?
- What is the purpose or meaning of a marriage or committed relationship?

Many people believe that having good sex is an important part of life, just like falling in love and having a strong relationship. Not enjoying sex or having sexual problems can be seen as a personal failing (e.g. "I am inadequate"), a relationship failing (e.g. "Not enough chemistry") or a partner's failing (e.g. "She is a starfish").

As a result of sexual problems, many people will either avoid sex, try to work on their sex life within the relationship they are in, or seek more satisfying sexual experiences outside of their current sexual relationship. Sexual difficulties are often believed to cause dissatisfaction and conflict in a relationship and believed to have the power to lead to the ending of the relationship if unresolved.

As such, having good sex in a committed relationship is seen by most as very important. There are strong cultural messages of marriage being the deathbed for desire, with the "spark" fading in a long-term relationship. However, because of the bounds of monogamy and cultural elevation of having a good sex life, sustaining a satisfying and positive sex life is commonly seen as one of the purposes of a marriage or committed relationship.

CHAPTER 6

THE HETERONORMATIVITY HYPE

One of the most insidious sexpectations is heteronormativity. Heteronormativity is the belief that it is normal for people to be one of two distinct and complementary genders (man or woman), be heterosexual, and follow a particular life pathway with specific gender-determined roles (marriage and babies, providers and caregivers, etc.). A heteronormative view therefore involves the alignment of biological sex, sexuality, gender identity and gender roles. Although some would say we have made great progress since the Sexual Revolution of the Sixties in terms of acceptance of gender and sexual diversity, heteronormativity is the reason same-sex-oriented people still have to "come out" – because it is assumed that they are straight until they do so.

GENDER BINARY AND GENDER ROLES

Gender binary is the practice of only recognising two distinct genders: man and woman. It is essential to heteronormativity because the scripted gender roles are based on the distinctions of man and woman. If the genders weren't opposite and completely separate, it would be much harder to define men as better in the business and provider roles and women as better in the domestic and caregiver roles.

From the moment that the nurses give female babies a pink blanket and male babies a blue blanket, expectations are set on us about how we should dress, feel, think, dream and be. Boys "should" play with cars and girls "should" play with dolls. Boys are more active and aggressive; girls are more gentle and kind. Boys are more spatial and girls more verbal. Boys use the men's public bathrooms and girls use the women's. A pilot is a man ... and I'll bet you pictured a female nurse in the description above!

Although there are some commonly found hormonal and brain development-related gender differences in young children, the differences are small and human brains cannot be categorised into two distinct classes of male brain or female brain (Joel et al., 2015). As such, most of these presumptions are rooted in heteronormativity and the behaviour and development that little boys and little girls show are largely due to "nurture": the environment they grow up in and life experiences they are encouraged to have.

If you identify as cisgender – where your personal identity corresponds with your birth sex – then you are, physically at least, in line with heteronormative expectations. You may, however, come into conflict with these expectations if you perform gender in a way that does not subscribe to the patriarchal gender roles or stereotypes of masculinity or femininity. For example, if you are a man who is not into ball-sports, cries in sad movies or wears high heels, or a woman who is a construction worker, shaves her head, or doesn't like children, you will more than likely have to justify or explain your preferences at some point in your life, and probably multiple times.

In response to this conflict with heteronormative expectations and the resulting rejection and ostracism they experience, some people choose to identify as "gender fluid" – not allowing themselves to be defined at either the male end or the female end of the gender spectrum. Some prefer to adopt a genderless identity, calling themselves "gender neutral". Transgender men and women identify as the gender opposite to the one they were assigned at birth because it better represents their identity.

> *'From as early as I can remember I've always felt different. I couldn't put my finger on exactly what it was, but I just didn't feel entirely like a boy. I was cross-dressing in my sister's clothes. I loved playing with her and her dolls. Eventually I went on the internet and typed in "boy feels like girl" and the result that came up was "transgender".'* – **Ashleigh**

Intersex people have anatomy or genetics that do not line up with typical expectations for either male or female people. Depending on the country and survey, approximately one in 1,500 or 2,000 births have atypical genitalia. A significant number of intersex people who have genital surgery during infancy are unhappy with it later in life – something that would be avoidable if not for the expectation of conforming to either male or female.

Very few of us question our gender assumptions. Gender is one of those sexpectations that get passed off as "normal" or "natural" and internalised as objective "truth". Therefore, particularly if we have a cisgendered identity, we may be vulnerable to minimising gender-dissonant parts of ourselves and being relatively gender-diversity insensitive when relating to other people. For example, a cisgendered man might suppress the desire to get a mani-pedi or make fun of himself when he gets one in an effort to excuse this gender-dissonant behaviour. Friends of this man may also ridicule and tease him for his well-groomed hands and feet.

The exception that proves the rule occurs with people who look stereotypically gender "queer". Because they look "queer", our heteronormative assumptions are broken and most people will be cautious of assuming their gender preference. However, just because someone looks like a "normal" guy, does not mean that they don't prefer to use the pronouns *she/her*.

Outside of gender-binary sexpectations we also get gender roles. Ideas of male and female roles are in every part of our culture. In the simple act of dining out we encounter them multiple times. Imagine you are a waiter at a prestigious restaurant serving a male and a female dining together. Who would you offer the wine list to? The bill? If you didn't know already, who would you guess ordered the steak and beer? And who the cocktail and salad? Even queer folk report that they experience gender-role assumptions placed on them because of their perceived masculinity or femininity.

'My partner usually gets the cheque placed in front of her – she is very androgynous-looking whereas I am more feminine. People think that because she looks like "the man" in the relationship she is the one that pays and makes all the financial decisions.' – **Cath**

EXERCISE: GENDER-BINARY SEXPECTATIONS
Which of these things do you associate with females and which with males?

Burping
Rescuing
Ballet
Emotional
Boxing
Flowers
Secretary
Shopping
Diamonds
Millionaire
Anger

Snoring
Finance
Nanny
Screwdriver
Garbage collector
Extreme sport
Facial
Leg hair
Handbag
Love songs

What interests, roles, feelings, clothes, activities and abilities do you have that are in line with the heteronormative expectations ascribed to your birth sex?

What interests, roles, feelings, clothes, activities and abilities do you have that are dissonant from the expectations ascribed to your birth sex?

How open are you with the parts of you that don't meet heteronormative expectations of your birth gender?

Have you ever felt shamed/pressured/judged in these areas?

Have you ever teased someone or made jokes at their expense for gender-dissonant behaviour or preferences?

If you are in a relationship, are you aware of falling into any "natural" gender roles around things such as the division of labour?

HETEROSEXUALITY

Content warning: There is a brief mention of sexual abuse with no explicit detail in this section.

We have come a long way in normalising same-sex attraction. Since 2001 when the Netherlands became the first country to legalise gay marriage, twenty-four countries have followed suit. Still, the number of countries where same-sex marriage is not legal outweighs the number of countries where it is. Gay-hate crimes and arrests are still in living memory for many older same-sex-attracted men and women, and even in the more progressive countries the assumption of heterosexuality is still deeply woven into the fabric of society.

Because under heteronormativity it is "abnormal" to be anything other than straight, those that come to identify in other ways will most likely have to deal with the automatic assumption that they are straight (particularly if they look stereotypically straight). By contrast, a straight couple would not have to explain their romantic involvement (although they may have to explain if they are *not* involved – more on this later).

'When I talk about my girlfriend, people just assume she is a female friend who I call a "girl friend". They act surprised, embarrassed or even offended when I correct that assumption.' – **Tracey**

Many people who are LGBT+ still speak about people discounting their experience by suggesting their sexuality is "just a phase" or that they are confused, or haven't found the right person yet. Many also speak about uncomfortable (and often intrusive) questions about how they "have sex".

There is also still very little representation of LGBT+ couples in the media, and when there is, it is highly stereotyped. LGBT+ individuals are rarely the main characters in movies and are often represented as visibly and behaviourally different from straight people. For example, gay men are often portrayed as "high camp", extravagant, flashy and promiscuous. Lesbian women are often portrayed as "butch", short-haired and man-hating.

However, despite their presentation in the media, LGBT+ people are decreasingly the minority. Same-sex attraction is more widely reported for millennials than older generations. In fact, fewer than half (46%) of millennials say they are completely heterosexual, according to new research from YouGov (2019). The Kinsey Scale, was created by Alfred Kinsey in 1948. It demonstrated that sexuality does not fit into two strict categories: homosexual and heterosexual but instead that sexuality is fluid and sexual behaviour is subject to change. Almost four in ten (38%) millennials describe themselves as being between one and six on the Kinsey Scale, meaning they are not completely heterosexual nor completely homosexual. Millennials are considerably more likely than Gen-Xers or Baby Boomers to describe themselves this way; just 25% of Gen-Xers and 15% of Baby Boomers say they are not completely heterosexual.

It is suggested that these changing attitudes say less about changing sexual orientations and more about how relatively unimportant it is today to define your identity based on sexual activity than it was three decades ago. When same-sex orientation and activity are seen as natural and healthy, it is no longer important to form a public identity based on sexual practices (Ambrosino, 2019).

TRENDS IN "CAMP"
(By James)

We have come a long way from the "hanky" code of the 1970s. Back then, when it was still dangerous to be open about your same-sex attraction, gay men would wear handkerchiefs or bandanas to indicate their sexual orientation and preference. Tied to the left – you are a top. On the right – a bottom. Then there were the colours, for instance: dark blue – anal sex; light blue – oral; grey – bondage; black – S&M; red – fisting; yellow – water sports … It was a veritable Morse code of signalling.

Since the Sexual Revolution, gay men have worn their preferences more freely, and have even created communities within the community. You have the "Bears" (usually hairy, larger guys) and "Twinks" (young, hairless, thin guys), who often socialise together. But then there are other sub-groups that come with their own labels but don't tend to have such created communities. There are "Twunks" (too old to be a Twink, but still physically the same attributes as a Twink), "Otters" (slim, taller guys with body hair), "Rice Queens" (guys into Asian guys), "Potato Queens" (Asian guys into white guys), etc.

Whilst these labels and communities do exist, the gay scene is becoming less segmented. There is more fluidity in how one identifies as gay – only a decade ago acting "camp" was out of fashion. Now gay male celebrities are wearing gowns and heels to the Met Gala. And it is looking like the gender- and sexual-preference signalling of old is giving way to unique personal expression and style preference without stereotypical and pigeonhole meaning attached. Who knows where we'll end up in the future, but looking at where we're heading, I'm up for it!

Even beyond identification, studies on human sexual arousal that measure pupil dilation (a sign of sexual arousal) and genital arousal show that women are on average physiologically sexually aroused to both male and female pornographic material. This means that regardless of how women self-reported their sexuality, their bodies responded positively to both hetero and homosexual sex (Rieger et al., 2016). Similar findings have been found, but to a lesser extent, for men. This led researchers to coin the category "mostly straight" and lends support to the idea of a sexuality continuum like the one that Kinsey proposed (Savin-Williams, 2017).

This capacity for women's bodily sexual arousal to be different to her self-report of subjective arousal has been studied since the 1970s. Researcher Meredith Chivers earned fame in 2009 when she found that heterosexual women's genitals became aroused when they viewed a bizarre range of sexual stimuli including the mating of bonobo apes! Yet, genital arousal is not a lie-detector test – arousal in a woman's body does not reveal what she really wants ... Otherwise by this research all women would be hankering for bonobo sex! It would also discredit the very common experience of men and women experiencing genital arousal in the context of sexual abuse.

'I didn't think of it as sexual assault for years because I had an orgasm, because I didn't try harder to stop it when it started to feel good ... Though I didn't want it to happen and I said no many times, I never went to the police because I felt they wouldn't believe me. I didn't realise that genital response can happen in reaction to sex-related cues, whether or not those cues are wanted or liked.' – **Stephanie**

How we choose to identify sexually does not necessarily represent our biological arousal patterns (sexual orientation), nor does our sexual identity always remain stable over time. Historically, people have dismissed sexual fluidity as a "phase" and this heteronormative assumption has led to demeaning terms such as "lesbians until graduation" (aka LUGS), suggesting that so-called people are going through a college "phase" of same-sex orientation and therefore their sexual preference is not to be taken seriously (Diamond, 2008).

A large longitudinal study indicated that stability of sexual orientation was more common than change when studied over a six-year period (Savin-Williams, Joyner & Rieger, 2012). However, sexual fluidity is also well documented; at some point in your life you could feel completely straight, whilst at other times, you might feel attracted to your same sex. Similar to studies discussed above on sexual arousal, this is more common in women than men identifying as heterosexual. It seems that "whereas sexual orientation in men appears to operate as a stable erotic 'compass', reliably channelling sexual arousal and motivation towards one gender or the other, sexual orientation in women does not appear to function in this fashion" (Diamond, 2012).

Social constructivist theories pose that sexual desire comes from cultural and psychosocial processes and that differences in male and female sexual fluidity are because men and women are socialised differently. Men are socially encouraged to get turned on by physical factors (boobs, nudity, lingerie, porn, etc.) and there is more prohibition for men to be same-sex oriented, whereas women are socially encouraged to sexually value sociocultural factors of love and intimacy (Baumeister, 2000). Moreover, women are also conditioned to be more emotionally expressive and intimate towards both males and females (Rust,

2000). However, the causal direction of this is unknown; female sexuality could be naturally more fluid leaving it more vulnerable to change from social learning, or social learning could cause female sexuality to develop to be less stable.

EXERCISE: SEXUAL ORIENTATION, IDENTITY AND FLUIDITY

Have you ever found yourself attracted to someone who is not of the gender you identify as sexually attracted to? How did you feel about and interpret that? Did you share that experience with anyone? What was their reaction?

Go online and find pictures of a very feminine-looking man and a very masculine-looking woman (preferably nude). Which do you find more attractive? If you were to define your sexuality based on being attracted to "masculinity" vs "femininity" (as opposed to men, women or both), how would you view yourself?

Have a look at our glossary. Are there any new terms there for you? Which of those terms do you relate to?

COUPLES PRIVILEGE AND THE RELATIONSHIP ESCALATOR

One of the most common ways I personally encounter heteronormativity in my day-to-day life is in the form of one simple question: 'Do you have a boyfriend?' This question is posed to me because I'm a woman, feminine-looking, and the common assumption is that women who look like me have either a boyfriend or a husband. Moreover, this type of questioning has become more frequent as I've got older. As a woman in my late thirties, public opinion is that if I'm not wearing a wedding ring or pushing a stroller by now, I should at least have a stable boyfriend – my "biological clock" is ticking after all!

In a heteronormative society, relationships exist in a hierarchy. That hierarchy puts middle-class and wealthy, heterosexual, cisgender, monogamous, married couples who have reproductive sex at the centre. All adult relationships are held up to this standard, and each step you take away from that standard, the less valuable your relationships are deemed by heteronormative society. So, for example, I am three steps away from the hierarchical goal: I am single, unmarried and I do not have reproductive sex. James is four steps away because he is also same-sex attracted.

In this heteronormative ideal, it is assumed a "couple" is the natural goal for everyone and results in a sort of "couple privilege" whereby these relationships are considered inherently more important and should be given priority over other types of relationships. As a single person I encounter this all the time: in my coupled friends having to ask their partner before agreeing to meet up with me; in being left out of invitations to couples' dinner parties and holidays; in being asked which of the men I'm dating I will "choose"; in someone seeing me with a male friend and asking me, 'Is anything happening there?'

The idea that a man and a woman can't be "just friends" (note that "just" indicates a lesser status for friendship) without romantic feelings developing is a part of couple privilege and also references the heteronormative concept of the Relationship Escalator. This concept refers to the expectation that a male–female relationship should go through a series of progressive steps towards the goal of a monogamous, cohabiting marriage – the "ideal" at the top of the escalator. It is the social standard by which most people determine whether a romantic, intimate or sexual connection is "serious" or "going anywhere".

'I broke up with my partner last month. We'd been together for two years and he still wasn't ready to take the next step and move in together. I know he loves me and we have fun together but if the relationship isn't going anywhere, I can't afford to waste my time. All my friends are married and pregnant with their first or second children now, and I feel I'm being left behind.' – **Jenny**

Most of us automatically and unconsciously adopt the Relationship Escalator as a roadmap for defining our goals for our relationships and lifestyle. Being brainwashed from childhood by fairy tales of "happily ever after", we evaluate our relationships and judge the relationships of others by these sexpectations. Just as we accept physical laws of nature such as the passing of time, the change of the seasons and that hot air rises, we accept that it is natural (even supernatural) to find "the one", fall in love, and for the development of the relationship to happen naturally along the Escalator pathway.

Couple privilege and the Relationship Escalator aren't only for heterosexual cisgendered people either. Transgender, genderqueer, lesbian, gay, bisexual and asexual people can all ride the Relationship Escalator and achieve a form of couple privilege too. In this way, the movement towards recognising same-sex marriage can be seen as supportive of the Escalator because it prioritises the pair bond as more socially important than the gender and sexual orientation of partners. Because of this, queer politics that resist heteronormativity calls for an abolition of government-sanctioned monogamy and instead wants the benefits given to married couples to be given to all people, regardless of relationship status.

'I've been with my partner for a few years now and people seemed shocked that we are not planning on moving in together when my

lease is up. Truth is, we rarely sleep over because his snoring keeps me awake … Although sometimes I feel it is weird and I worry about where we are heading, I don't see why we should have to do the whole cohabiting thing ' – **Ben**

Getting to the top of the Escalator validates you as an adult and as worthy of love and respect. If you don't get there – or don't want to ride at all – there is a chance you will be labelled as immature, damaged, selfish and untrustworthy. As such, couple privilege is also built on singlism – prejudice against single people (De Paulo, 2011). Above the age of around twenty-five, single people are often presumed to be inferior, difficult, flawed, less stable or valid, less important and more obliged to accommodate than people who are in a couple because they haven't conformed to the couple sexpectation.

The steps in the Relationship Escalator are one-way with no provision for taking a break and stepping off or going back down the Escalator without breaking up. Similarly, relationships that linger too long in an intermediate phase are deemed "dead ends".

The steps have been summarised by Amy Garhan (2017) as:

1. **Making contact**: flirting, dating and possibly sex.
2. **Initiation**: romantic courtship and emotional investment, aka "falling in love".
3. **Claiming and defining**: Declaration of reciprocated love, agreements of sexual monogamy, presenting in public as a couple and adoption of relationship labels, for example, "my boyfriend", and agreements of sexual monogamy.
4. **Establishment**: Setting patterns for spending time together and mutual accountability for whereabouts and behaviour.

5. **Commitment**: Moving in together, sharing property or finances, getting engaged.
6. **Conclusion**: Getting married. The relationship is now "finalised" and the structure is expected to remain static until one partner dies.
7. **Legacy**: Buying a home, having kids. These are often deemed less crucial to the Escalator experience than a few decades ago but some couples may still not feel fully "valid" until they achieve this.

Couples that succeed to make it to the top of the Escalator enjoy social and legal privileges. Reflecting the couple privilege inherent in modern-day Western society, they enjoy tax advantages, legal protections for joint property, survivorship benefits, insurance benefits, social security benefits in the United States, even package holidays are made with couples in mind. Couples that do not make it to the top, don't stay at the top or individuals who don't get on it at all are assumed to have personal problems, relationship problems or bad luck: for most people, it is not a question of whether there might be a problem with the idea of the Relationship Escalator and the social construction of the "couple" itself, but rather with those who don't adhere to it.

If a couple reaches the establishment phase of the Escalator and then breaks up – as the majority of committed relationships now do – the relationship is deemed as "failed" despite whatever good was achieved during its lifespan or whatever affection, support or friendship may persist afterwards. Our culture does not have any models to transition or conclude romantic relationships well, and divorce and break-ups are usually stressful and traumatic for all involved as a result. It is often the pain and disillusionment that occurs when the Relationship Escalator fails to deliver the "happily ever after" it promises, that leads people to question monogamy and normative relationship models.

'We became non-monogamous after being together for seven years. We reached this point where we loved each other and didn't want to separate but also felt dissatisfied in life and stuck. When we spoke to friends about non-monogamy, we alienated a lot of people. They couldn't grasp that we could both be okay with the idea of each other having other relationships.' – **Dave**

WHAT IS OFF THE ESCALATOR BUT ON THE TABLE?

Although alternative examples of relationships are less prevalent and gain almost no media attention, there are plenty of non-Escalator options out there. These include:

- Single people who value ongoing relationships but don't want to get married or live with a partner
- Polyamorous people who believe in having more than one loving, intimate relationship at a time, with everyone involved having knowledge and consent (aka "ethical non-monogamy")
- People who don't believe that relationships should be bound by rules except those that the individuals involved mutually agree upon, including the rules prioritising romantic or sexual relationships above other relationships (aka "relationship anarchy")

- People who have a different life-focus such as their work, studies, art, hobbies, children and so on, who can't or don't want to give a relationship the time that the Escalator-style relationships typically require
- Swingers who consensually engage in recreational sex beyond their primary partnership
- People who desire emotional intimacy or life partnership that does not involve sex and/or romance (aka asexual, ace, grey-A, aromantic, or queer platonic)
- BDSM/kink relationships involving intimate power-exchange dynamics that may or may not be sexual and which may involve people other than their primary partner
- Long-distance relationships. For example, when a partner is deployed in the military or physically unavailable for long periods that therefore have implicit or explicit allowances for additional relationships
- People who use the services of sex workers
- People who prefer to "hook up", where there is no expectation of commitment, be it in a friends-with-benefits scenario or with a new acquaintance.

Interestingly, cheating forms a *part* of the Escalator and couple-privilege structure. It is because of the assumptions of monogamy and relationship progression, that cheating is called cheating, and is concealed and shameful. If we didn't have the step of committing to sexual exclusivity so early in the Escalator journey, and if there were provisions for going back down or stepping off the Escalator, perhaps someone who found themselves attracted to another partner – or had a drunken unplanned infidelity – would feel safer openly discussing it. Many people who are unfaithful do not cheat maliciously, and many still hold a lot of love for their committed partner and desire to remain within their relationship. Often what keeps them from being open and honest about infidelity is the real threat of traumatising their partner, as well as the threat that this will cause the end of the relationship. Both outcomes can be seen to result from most people's unconsciously held sexpectations, monogamy and the Relationship Escalator.

EXERCISE: HAPPILY EVER AFTER

Think back to when you were a child. What did you think your future would hold in terms of relationships?

Have you had a period of being single as an adult? Do you remember any experiences which you might now categorise as "singlism" or "couple privilege" at work?

Have you ever had a relationship go "off-track"? What explanation did you have for that?

If you are in a monogamous Relationship Escalator-type relationship, how would you feel if progress stopped or if your partner asked to step back down the Escalator (e.g. move out but still remain in the relationship)?

Where would you say you are on the below scale of sexual exclusivity? Have you been at a different point on the spectrum in the past or can you imagine being so in the future?

Scale of Sexual Exclusivity

MONOSEXUAL

Monogamous – it's not acceptable to hug, kiss or flirt with anyone other than your partner.

Open to your partner watching porn or other types of sexy stimulus but not with another real person.

Monogam-ish – it's okay to snog another person or do certain sexual activities but not others. (Note: There might be rules around this, e.g. 'Don't ask, don't tell', 'Only with a sex worker', 'Only when you are travelling overseas', 'Only with someone of a certain gender', 'Never with the same person twice'.)

Swinging or open relationships.

Polyamorous people who have multiple partners (sexual and non-sexual) and romantic relationships.

POLYSEXUAL

CHAPTER 7

THE CHEMISTRY CONUNDRUM

LOVE AT FIRST SIGHT

It's not a huge leap to see that choosing a long-term partner is, for many people, about sex. When our culture elevates the concept of monogamy and the Relationship Escalator, we are essentially choosing the person we are going to have sex with "till death do us part".

So, what sexpectations influence how we choose that partner?

In a world where dating often requires a lot of work, falling in love at first sight has a strong appeal. We've all heard the stories of two strangers locking eyes in the supermarket cereal aisle, feeling a jolt of electricity and an unexplainable sense of recognition, knowing they found "the one". Many of us will have our own stories or have heard friends who talk about falling in love at first sight and research suggests that as many as 60% of people report experiencing this at some time (Naumann, 2004).

We live in a culture where feeling attraction and desire as well as falling in love are deemed a prerequisite for committing to a romantic/sexual relationship and plenty of people will wait years to experience this feeling, foregoing several very suitable prospective partners in its pursuit. In general, we are becoming more and more open to "casual sex", but we still hold out to feel that chemistry and fall in love before committing to a long-term sexual relationship.

'Many, many girls can pass the "hook-up" standard. If you're reasonably attractive, not a total bore, and interested, sure. However, dating means commitment. You are throwing away an unknown amount of pussy of unknown quality. So if a man can find sexual satisfaction whilst single, the cost-benefit analysis of a relationship is pretty uneven. In order for the perceived benefits to outweigh the perceived costs, the girl in question needs to be an absolute no-brainer. You've got to be a total package – I've got to feel that special something about you to even consider it.' – **Dan**

Feeling "chemistry" or "love at first sight" hasn't always been such an important sexpectation when choosing a committed sexual relationship. Alternative models such as arranged marriages have historically been common in many cultures and there are a number of regions where this custom continues today. In these arrangements, a couple commits to each other on political, financial or religious grounds and not because of attraction, romantic love or sexual passion.

Research has shown that love at first sight is highly correlated with attraction – the more physically attractive you perceive someone, the greater chance you'll feel love at first sight (Zsok, 2017). However, physical attraction has also been shown to be more than skin deep. Other factors that influence our sense of someone's attractiveness include: pheromones, the sound of one's voice (deep in men, higher pitched in women), wearing the colour red (on women), propinquity (the frequency of interaction), familiarity, perceived similarity (in bone structure, personality, attitudes, background, life goals and physical appearance), positive personality traits (like kindness, agreeableness, etc.), and reciprocal liking (if you think someone is attracted to you).

> *'When we first met, I never saw Liam as all that attractive. I was with someone else at the time and I remember reassuring him that Liam and I were just friends and I would never be into him in that way! I meant it too! It was only a few years later when we found ourselves single at the same time that other feelings grew. I'd always admired Liam's intelligence and loved how similar our views were on some things. But I also started picking up on things I'd never noticed before – his gorgeous blue-green eyes, the way he walked … All. His. Muscles! The morning I woke up from a sexy dream with Liam as the leading man, I knew things had changed for me.'*
> **– Meg**

This list of other factors has implications for dating in the digital age where people are dismissed with the swipe of a finger based mainly on the superficial information one can glance in a few photos. Given that we can develop attraction based on many other non-physical factors, in swiping left we may be unnecessarily limiting our possibilities. Furthermore, our preoccupation with more superficial physical attractiveness – as promoted through pornography, celebrity culture, social media and image-altering technology – can have large negative effects on our self-esteem and body image. It can also lead to a raft of sexual problems when people become self-conscious in their nudity, or overly dependent on the visual appeal of their partner for their turn-on.

> 'When we first started dating, I was really into him. We had huge chemistry. Now it's been a few years, and we are engaged, but he's put on a lot of weight and although I know it's superficial, I just don't find him attractive anymore. I never feel like having sex with him and I don't know if we should begin a marriage on that basis …' – **Kate**

Research has also shown that there are plenty of factors that predict long-term satisfying sexual relationships, and attraction isn't one of them! Pre-eminent couples researcher and therapist John Gottman has investigated what leads to long-term happy relationships and found that the most successful couples are the ones who worked for their relationships in the two areas of building something meaningful together, and interacting well together (Gottman & Silver, 2000). This means it's not looks, lightning bolts or "chemistry" that will result in the perfect mate – it's how skilful you both are at communicating, sustaining a friendship and supporting each other. We can begin to understand then why choosing a sexual partner to commit to is better done with your head and not further south!

So, with all the research pointing in the other direction, why are we still so seduced by attraction and "chemistry" as essential ingredients in our romantic and sexual relationships? Why do we gobble up romantic comedies and hold "falling in love" in such high regard? Why do women, and increasingly men, spend large amounts of money on diets, exercise regimes, clothes, shoes, makeup, Botox, fillers, cosmetic surgery, etc. all in the service of making ourselves more attractive?

LOVE IS A DRUG AND A DELUSION

To my mind, the answer lies in a combination of two things: brain chemicals and the "halo effect". It is a fact that we are both chemically and cognitively biased towards physical attractiveness – it's in our biology. However, I am *not* suggesting that we shouldn't want to be attracted to a potential sexual or romantic partner. Rather, we need to be aware of the "attraction trap" and not romanticise finding someone hot or having "chemistry". Enjoy it, but don't make decisions based on it. The relationship between attraction and love is unlikely to be linear or causal: attraction (at first sight) does not necessarily lead to love; affection and love can lead to attraction; and neither attraction nor feelings of love necessarily predicts sexual or relationship satisfaction.

When you begin to fall in love, your brain releases a predictable cocktail of chemicals that result in the euphoric feeling that most people associate with early love (now known as New Relationship Energy (NRE)). This same chemical "high" is interpreted by some as a spiritual experience of the "soulmate". The chemicals of dopamine, serotonin and oxytocin make falling in love feel amazing; they lead to increased energy, less need for sleep or food, more focused attention and obsession, delight in the small details of the new person, as well as feelings of excitement, wellbeing and happiness.

Adrenaline, oestrogen (in women) and testosterone, also released when we fall in love, increase the perceived attractiveness of a prospective partner. It has been proven that we can find someone more attractive just because we are in situations where adrenaline is artificially heightened (e.g.

on a rickety bridge) (Dutton & Aron, 1974) or a rollercoaster (Meston & Frohlich, 2003). This phenomenon of mistaking anxiety or raised adrenaline as excitement and sexual attraction is known as the "misattribution of arousal". It reveals how easily our perception of attractiveness and sexual appeal can be influenced.

'I always fell for "bad boys" – the ones that were dangerous, unpredictable, moody. They'd cancel on me, get drunk and booty call me, disappear for weeks on end only to message me out of the blue again like nothing had happened. It was only when my therapist pointed out that the excitement I felt was probably more likely anxiety from walking on eggshells around them that the penny dropped.' – **Jessie**

It's not just danger that will get us all excited. The qualities of a new relationship, including novelty and unpredictability, will also cause anxiety and adrenaline. As such, the low desire and low sexual attraction many experience in long-term relationships may come about because of the greater mundanity in your life, greater knowledge of your partner and a sense of safety in your relationship. As Esther Perel writes: "There is a powerful tendency in long-term relationships to favour the predictable over the unpredictable. Yet, without an element of uncertainty, there is no longing, no anticipation, no frisson" (2006).

So much emphasis is put on being attracted to our sexual partners. We have all had the experience of being "into" someone and "just not feeling it" with another. We tend to assume that someone's attractiveness is therefore a necessary ingredient of any romantic or sexual connection. But when attraction has been shown to have as much to do with the situation we meet someone in (and the adrenaline released)

WHAT IS "CHEMISTRY" REALLY?

When people talk about "chemistry" they are not far wrong! Romantic love is probably better viewed as an addiction, rather than an emotion. Everything that occurs when we find ourselves "into" someone is because of the chemicals released in our brain. The process generally happens like this:

1. It is possible that we pick up pheromones and cues about our sexual partner's immune system through scent, which helps us determine whether we are suitable for one another. This is thought to begin the process of initial desire.

2. Oestrogen in women and testosterone in men and women is released to make us feel attracted and drawn to our sexual partner and these hormones increase our sexual desire and energy levels.

3. Dopamine is released to make us feel good. Dopamine is associated with motivation and goal-directed behaviour, hence the drive to pursue our sexual partner. It increases novelty – our partner seems exciting and special to us. It gives us a sense of joy; our world becomes brighter, details more sharp; we are emboldened; we feel more capable and creative; and memories are more easily made.

4. Adrenaline makes us interested. We achieve high levels of attention, attraction and energy; our thinking seems clearer; we are more aware, more awake, more focused and more responsive. We lose the need for sleep or food. Our heart beats faster, our palms

become sweaty, we get butterflies in our stomach and our pupils dilate (the "come-hither" look).

5.   After we leave our sexual partner, serotonin levels drop, which leaves us obsessing over them. The more we obsess, the more likely we are to seek them out again. Serotonin increases again when we have sex, producing an addictive cycle.

6.   Oxytocin, referred to as the "love hormone", and vasopressin are released in response to physical touch such as hugging, kissing and sex. These hormones enhance the monogamous bond between sexual partners and help develop a strong attachment.

as it does with the person we are attracted to, we might be better off spending our money on extreme sports rather than extreme makeovers!

A person's attractiveness has also been found to produce a cognitive bias known as the "Halo Effect" (Thorndyke, 1920). When we find someone attractive, we are more inclined to think positively of them in other areas, even when we know very little about them.

This effect has been extensively studied, and attractiveness has been found to influence people's judgements of someone's personality, intelligence, kindness, trustworthiness, friendliness and life success, to name just a few! For example, in one early study, more attractive people were judged by strangers as having more socially desirable personality traits, they were assumed to lead happier lives, have happier marriages, have more career success and hold more secure and prestigious jobs (Dion, Berscheid & Walster, 1972).

There seems to be a reciprocal effect where qualities such as positive personality traits (like kindness, agreeableness, etc.) make someone more attractive. Further to this, studies show that even if you have never met a person but perhaps seen a picture and you find them attractive, you will assume they have positive traits because of the Halo Effect! However, we'd better hope our "love-blinded" biases are proven true in the long term because couples are more likely to be satisfied in their relationship and less likely to break up when a partner's actual personality characteristics match those we envision an ideal mate to have (Zentner, 2005).

Although our society has put high emphasis on physical attraction, love at first sight and chemistry, all is not what it seems. No matter which way you slice it, when you find someone attractive you are *less* likely to accurately judge their personal qualities. A brain in love is a brain on drugs. Like drugs of the illegal variety, this "chemistry" makes us feel good and alters our perceptions around attractiveness. And attractiveness in itself leads to bias. Moreover, physical attraction is a multifaceted concept that goes far beyond the physical, therefore love at first *sight* is a misnomer at best, and the basis for a poor relationship choice at worst.

IS HE GAY ... OR EUROPEAN? BY JAMES

For decades, gay culture has been entwined with fashion, fitness and fabulousness. Gay men have always been seen at gallery openings, fashion shows and the latest musical premieres, not just because it's what we were into, but most likely because it's where we felt most welcomed and protected.

Although we are now more free to explore less traditionally "gay" scenes, unfortunately the mindset that gay men should look like one of Madonna's backing dancers remains. As does gay gym culture and the gay party scene, which can often be likened to an underwear photoshoot or a porn set. Although not all gay men are into the circuit scene, this culture has spread deep into the gay psyche.

The unattainable beauty standards of the gay culture can be seen to be related to our perception around masculinity and "coming-out" trauma. For a long time, being gay was associated with being a sissy, weak and feminine. A large percentage of gay males grow up feeling detached, dismissed and rejected by their male peers. Building our body can be a way of proving we are strong, masculine and belong with the guys.

The masculine ideal is lean, fit and muscular and good at physical activities – think of a sports star. But this attitude to achieve such physical perfection has shown to have devastating effects on mental health. (Chaney, 2008) Whilst some ideas of what it means to be masculine have changed in the past five to ten years, the ideal of physical perfection continues. When dating, gay men are critical both of their own appearance but also the attractiveness of the other guy. Across the gay chatrooms and apps the common phrase can be read: "No fems, no fats, no …"

It doesn't just stop at general attractiveness either; pictures of disembodied cocks are sent out freely for pre-hook-up assessment. We talk about each other's physical features and place excessive value on the body parts that we find most attractive. Is it any wonder that gay men are thought to only represent 5% of the total male population but among men who have eating disorders, 42% identify as gay (Frederick

& Essayli, 2016)? Gay men report significantly more body dissatisfaction, drive for thinness and drive for muscularity than heterosexual men. Unsurprisingly, lesbian women report similar pressures and body dissatisfaction as heterosexual women, with the exception of increased drive for muscularity (Yean et al., 2013).

EXERCISE: JUST NOT THAT INTO YOU

Have you ever dated or hooked up with anyone you liked and thought would be a good partner but felt you couldn't pursue a relationship because you didn't have the chemistry you craved? Has anyone said this to you?

Have you ever experienced intense chemistry with a "bad boy" or a "drama queen", where there was a lot of anxiety or drama (and hence adrenaline) in the relationship, making this person seem more attractive?

Has all your great sex been with people you felt an intense attraction to? Have you ever had great sex with someone who wasn't your traditional "type"?

When you have found chemistry, experienced love at first sight or been really attracted to a person and had the opportunity to have a relationship with them, how long did these feelings last for you?

When you have had a successful long-term relationship, what would you say made the relationship successful? How much of the success would you put down to your initial attraction or chemistry?

CHAPTER 8

THE LIBIDO LIES

LUST AND PASSION

Just like we have a view that "first comes love, then comes marriage", we have a view that in the proper order, first comes desire, then comes sex – you should want to have sex before having it. Most people think that desire should be spontaneous, because this is the only way we ever see desire portrayed on TV, in the movies, and in porn ... Couples are just going about their days when all of a sudden a lightning bolt of sexual desire hits and they are swept up in the throes of passion.

These ideas may have come into being following the pioneering work on the human sexual response cycle by Masters, Johnson and Kaplan in the 1960s and 1970s. The traditional model of the human sexual response cycle based on their work suggests an initial stage of desire leading on to arousal after which there is a period of heightened arousal, which peaks briefly before falling away to resolution after the release of orgasm (Kaplan, 1979).

The presence of sexual thoughts, fantasies and an innate urge to experience sexual tension and release have traditionally been considered the markers of desire (Kaplan, 1979). However, in one study 97% of women and 60% of men reported having engaged in sexual behaviour in the absence of desire (Beck et al., 1991). In fact, research has found that both men and women have many varied reasons for engaging in sex other than desire. These include to increase emotional closeness, to share physical pleasure, to feel attractive, to improve sex skills, to feel masculine/feminine amongst 237 other reasons (Meston & Buss, 2007).

Moreover, for women and men, desire can follow arousal rather than precede it, meaning that some people have to be involved in sexual activity before they desire it (Basson, 2000). This "responsive desire" is thought to be the primary desire style for roughly 30% of women, and 5% of men and most people experience a period of it at some point in their lives (Nagoski, 2015).

A SMORGASBORD OF LIBIDOS

Dr Sandra Pertot (2007) has defined a veritable buffet of libido types to help people understand how they tick, and to normalise that not everyone is prone to being caught up in the throes of passion like you see in the movies. These "types" not only reflect different biological drives but also the different sexual attitudes and sexpectations held by some people. Although I imagine that there are far more "types" than she lists, her work emphasises that often reality varies from our cultural sexpectations of passion-fuelled love making.

Sensual Type
Use sex to feel connected

'I don't care about sexual gymnastics as much as I care about my partner being present and emotionally available.'

Erotic Type
Want steamy sex and believe sex is a high priority (the cultural norm)

'Sex is only good if it's passionate and intense.'

Dependent Type
Rely on sex as stress relief

'I need sex to cope with my life.'

Entitled Type
Place a lot of value on getting their desires met.

'I deserve to get what I want in the bedroom.'

Addictive Type
Find it hard to turn down sex and can cheat as a result

'I can't resist any opportunity to have sex.'

Reactive Type
Make sex all about their partner's needs.

'Pleasing my partner gets me hot under the collar.'

Stressed Type
Feel performance pressure and anxiety around sex

'I want sex, but I steer clear because I worry I can't please my partner.'

Disinterested Type

Not into sex, perhaps asexual

> *'I wouldn't care if I never had sex again.'*

Detached Type

Feel desire but only interested in solo sex (e.g. after a betrayal)

> *'I'd rather be masturbating.'*

Compulsive Type

Specific fetishes or fantasies are needed to feel desire

> *'I need to have [fill in the blank] in order to get turned on.'*

So, the situation is that beyond the adrenaline- and dopamine-fuelled six to eighteen-month "honeymoon period" of New Relationship Energy (which puts everyone's libido into hyper-drive), a large proportion of women and some men will rarely feel desire before engaging in sexual activity. Add to that pre-existing sexpectations – such as marathon sessions of sexual acrobatics ending in mutual orgasm. Then, throw in the desire-dampening effect of stress, physical health problems, fatigue, the demands of children, mental health problems and tension in the relationship (to name just a few), it is a wonder that long-term couples even have sex at all, let alone passion-fuelled fuck fests!

> *'We have three kids and live in a small house. I work two jobs. She works one. We both team up to take care of the housework and running the kids to this and that activity. But besides not having the time or energy, we're in our forties and my wife has become less*

interested in having sex. We haven't had sex in a couple of years but not a day goes by that we don't hug and kiss each other and say, "I love you."' – **Tyrone**

Yet, how many people have felt hurt, confused, abandoned, frustrated, angry and betrayed when they find that their partner no longer wants to rip their clothes off? It is easy for some people to take it personally and doubt their attractiveness, or begin to distrust their partner and worry that they are getting their sexual needs met elsewhere. Until recently, few Hollywood movies featured honest depictions of what happens to the passionately in-love couple after they say, 'I do'. As such, many of us have no script for correctly interpreting loss of desire or the emergence of responsive desire, and even less idea of how to build a satisfying sex life when this happens.

'I'm attracted to my wife, and would love to be intimate with her at least once a week. But my wife would probably go six to twelve months or more without reaching towards me. Having to "make the move" every time, in a hundred different sensitive ways is exhausting and works away at your own self-esteem. You wonder what it is about you that is so fundamentally unattractive.'
– **Edmond**

DESIRE DISCREPANCY

More often than not in a relationship, there is one partner who has a higher drive and desire for sex than the other. Stereotypically we usually think of men as having higher drives but this is not always the case. This leads to a "desire discrepancy" and the "pursuer-distancer" cycle (King, 1997).

In this cycle, the partner with the higher drive pursues the low-drive partner for sex. When his/her overtures and requests are continually rebuffed, the pursuer can become angry or despondent. He/she may withdraw and become emotionally distant in the relationship. Alternatively, the lower-drive partner may feel frustrated or guilty and give in and have "mercy sex". The lower-drive distancer may even become reluctant to engage in non-sexual affection such as hugging or kissing for fear it will lead their partner on. Both scenarios generate resentment and contempt in the relationship.

'He doesn't pressure me, but I pressure myself – I feel I can't win. I'm having to stop myself from avoiding sitting next to him on the couch, in case it gives him ideas. I either feel guilty for not having sex, or I feel guilty and like a bad feminist for having sex when I don't feel like it.' – **Sarah**

Despite desire discrepancy and loss of passion being an almost ubiquitous occurrence, many couples are resistant to the standard advice to schedule time to be sexual and "work" at better sex. They cling on to the myth, the sexpectation, that desire should be spontaneous and that if it doesn't happen naturally, someone is being disingenuous.

The interesting thing about these arguments is that even in the peak honeymoon period of the early stages of dating, sex is still planned, just in a different way. When we are dating someone we set … dates! We may know days or even weeks in advance that sex might be on offer. So, most people are probably resisting the implication of sex without desire – that the sex is not the result of an uncontrollable hunger for one another sexually – more than the idea of scheduling sex.

Similarly, many people resist sexual bartering in a relationship because it assumes the desire for sex is absent. Sexual bartering, also called "choreplay" is when we agree to have sex in exchange for some other thing (e.g. a special favour). For men, having to "earn" sexual privileges rather than having them passionately and freely given can be perceived as a power play, manipulative and humiliating. For women, sexual bartering can seem a bit too close to prostitution because the perceived focus is on the outcome of the act (the "payment") rather than the act itself.

'It stopped being fun after thirty years of marriage. She never initiated, and I got the feeling she was only doing it to get something she wanted, or to cover up something she did. That feeling of being played just kills you inside.' – **Trevor**

Unfortunately our beliefs about desire and passion can have a real effect on the success of our relationships. Studies have shown that low passion is linked to low commitment, particularly if you have the sexpectation that passion cannot be reignited (Carswell & Finkel, 2018). In other words, if we believe that once passion is lost, it's gone for good, then once we experience low passion we are more likely to end the relationship.

BUT DOES PASSION ALWAYS FADE?

Besides the sexpectations that we should feel attraction and "chemistry" for our partner and that desire is a prerequisite for sex, we are also led to believe that passion fades in the long term. It is thought that humans habituate to pleasure – a process known as "hedonic adaptation" – and studies have shown that the same sexy stimulus (e.g. a particular fantasy or erotic image) ceases to produce the same arousal with repetition over time (O'Donohue & Plaud, 1991).

All relationships naturally experience ebbs and flows in sexual passion. However, this can be weathered by couples for whom other relationship aspects are going strong (Birnbaum & Finkel, 2015). In fact, a 2011 survey found that 40% of respondents who had been married for ten years or longer reported being "very intensely in love". The things that contributed to this love were thinking positively about the partner and thinking about the partner when apart, affectionate behaviours and sexual intercourse, shared novel and challenging activities, and general life happiness (O'Leary et al., 2011). Of course, we don't know how these people defined "love", and if they would say the love they felt was as passionate as it was in the early stages of the relationship, but the results are still encouraging!

Similarly, brain scans of people who reported still being intensely and passionately in love after being married for at least ten years showed that, just as with people newly in love, the "dopamine-reward system" part of the brain still lit up when they looked at photos of their spouse. Indeed, there was just one important difference between them and new lovers: amongst the older lovers, brain regions associated with anxiety were no longer active, instead, there was activity in the areas associated with calmness. (Acevedo et al., 2012). As such, it has been proposed that intense romantic love (with intensity, engagement and sexual desire) can exist in some long-term relationships, but without the obsessive component common in the early stages of love (Acevedo & Aron, 2009).

Many theories have been proposed that New Relationship Energy and the "bubble" of new love gives way to a more mature, companionate love and glossy magazines are full of tips on how to "reignite" the spark. Yet, there is some (albeit small) evidence to suggest that at least some people have kept the passion in their relationship alive … If this is biologically possible, perhaps the concept of the marital "deathbed" may also be a spurious, culturally endorsed sexpectation.

'I've been with my partner for six years and we still have the "spark". It never went away. We fuck at least once a day and like to surprise each other with little gifts and notes. I think it's important to never stop chasing your partner. A lot of it is chemistry and compatibility, but much of it is also choice. To keep things going, you have to consistently choose your partner, and make them feel special and desired.' – **Ted**

A QUESTION OF CONSENT

The prevalence of passion fading and people not desiring sex but engaging in it anyway has implications for the notion of consent. Some would say that a person saying yes to sex for reasons other than sexual excitement (e.g. out of fear of relationship breakdown if they did not consent) are not truly consenting, even more so if we use the notion of "enthusiastic consent" as our consent goal post.

How we define consent – legally and culturally – has come a long way in recent years. It used to be that a person had to say no if they weren't consenting. The "enthusiastic consent" model encourages people to make sure the person they're about to have sex with is enthusiastic about the sexual interaction and wants to be there. Enthusiasm is seen as important because "enthusiasm – the unmistakable sense of not being able to keep your hands off each other [in an encounter] – [...] is harder to mistake for anything else" (Hinsliff, 2015). This is an extension of the "yes means yes" model, which is the "free verbal or non-verbal communication of a feeling of willingness to engage in sexual activity" (Hickman & Muehlenhard, 1999).

The "enthusiastic consent" model has been criticised by asexual people and sex workers because people in these categories may choose to have sex with people even though they are not "particularly wanting it or enjoying it themselves" (Zheng, 2014). Additionally there are plenty of consenting adults that may be willing to have sex, such as couples who want to fall pregnant or couples who want to please each other, but may not necessarily want to or feel able to summon the ardour required for "enthusiasm" (Ross, 2015).

EXERCISE: WHEN THE HONEYMOON IS OVER
What are some of your reasons to have sex other than passion/desire? Circle those that you relate to and feel free to add your own.

Physical Reasons

- Exercise
- Pleasure
- Warmth

- Attraction to a person
- Stress relief
- To reduce sex drive
- To burn excess energy
- To feed "skin hunger" (need for touch)

Emotional Reasons

- To feel loved by a partner
- To show a partner you love them
- An expression of commitment
- Gratitude for something that was done
- To boost mood or relieve depression
- To foster jealousy
- To feel nurturance and taken care of
- Because you are angry
- For affection and closeness
- Sexual curiosity
- To relieve boredom (procrastinate)
- To reinforce your masculinity/femininity
- To feel "normal"

Goal-Based Reasons

- To make a baby
- Spiritual transcendence
- To improve reputation or social status
- To "fit in"
- To seek revenge
- To make money
- To get to sleep
- To resolve an argument

- In a sexual bartering agreement
- To comply to a schedule/routine
- To have an orgasm
- To improve your sex skills
- To distract yourself from other things
- To put your partner in a good mood
- To learn more about yourself
- To heal wounds from the past
- To show someone how skilful you are

Insecurity Reasons

- To boost self-esteem
- To feel attractive
- To keep a partner faithful
- Out of a feeling of duty
- To relieve peer pressure
- To relieve pressure from partner
- Enhancement of power or identity
- Experiencing the power of one's partner
- To prevent losing a relationship

Keeping in mind that any partner will have his or her own reasons for having sex (not necessarily to do with lust or wanting pleasure or orgasm), how would knowing their reasons change how you might "do" sex? How might you discuss your intentions for this sex beforehand?

Have you experienced the passion fading in a longer-term relationship? Did you expect this to happen? Is there variation in your experience of passion in different relationships for you, or was it pretty similar across all of them? If there is variation, what do you make of that?

Have you had an experience with a partner who has a much *lower* sex drive than you? How did you interpret their lack of interest? How did you cope with the variation between you in the relationship?

Have you ever had an experience with a partner who has a much *higher* sex drive than you? How did you interpret their need for sex? How did you cope with the variation between you in the relationship?

What would it mean to you to have a sexless relationship?

How do you feel about scheduling sex or sexual bartering? Why?

CHAPTER 9

THE HOMO SAPIEN HORNDOG

MEN WANT SEX

Alex snuggles up and begins caressing Jules' arm suggestively. Jules lets out a small sigh and pulls away. Alex is frustrated and says, 'We haven't had sex in two weeks. You're not in the mood again?' and then stomps off to another room to watch TV. Jules feels guilty and ashamed, but just doesn't feel like it and can't force it. The couple goes to bed feeling sad and disconnected again.

Who is the man or woman in this scenario? There is a common sexpectation that men have high libidos and always want sex, so you would be forgiven for thinking that Alex was a man and Jules was a woman. It is a widely held belief, even amongst scientists, that males are naturally promiscuous whilst females are coy and choosy.

The male libido is typically viewed as an innate, automatic, animalistic drive, always ready to be aroused. Tied to this, it is commonly assumed that sex is a biological imperative for men, like hunger; that men will initiate sex; have a strong "sex drive"; be sexually skilled; they will not refuse sex if offered it; seek multiple partners; that they "only want one thing" and will pursue recreational or "no-strings" sex over relationships (Masters et al., 2013; Pham, 2016).

The evolutionary hypothesis explaining this dates back to Charles Darwin and from these roots, grew the theory of "parental investment" (Trivers, 1972). It suggested that because there is relatively low energy expenditure and investment in producing sperm, men have evolved to abandon their mate and indiscriminately seek other females for mating, so they can spread their seed far and wide, ensuring the survival of their genes. In contrast, because pregnancy and child-rearing are difficult and energetically expensive, women approach sex differently. They need a man who will stay by them and their young and care for them.

In line with this, traditional sexual scripts see women as being desired but not desiring sex, having weak sex drives, resisting advances, and being more highly valued if they are less sexually experienced. They are seen as preferring romance and sex within the context of a relationship, wanting commitment and monogamy, and seeking emotional intimacy and trust with sex (Masters et al., 2013).

Although recent studies have shown some evidence of movement away from these gendered sexpectations, these sexual scripts still very much influence our sex lives today, even when the evolutionary explanations have been all but disproven (Snowdon, 1997). For example, it comes as little surprise to most people that men have been found to be more likely to use dating apps like Tinder for casual sex (Carpenter & McEwan, 2016) and are less selective in their choices than women (Tyson et al., 2016). Similarly, there remains an assumption in longer-term relationships that sex plays an important role in male fidelity ("give him sex or else he'll go elsewhere for it") and, indeed, research has found that men, more so than women, cite that they cheated for reasons of sexual desire – feeling unsatisfied with the sex in a relationship and wanting something new (Selterman et al., 2017).

But are these gendered sexpectations a social construction or do they represent biological fact?

A review on literature in the field performed in 2001 confirmed that on average, men do report desiring sex more than women. Men were found to have more spontaneous thoughts about sex; more frequent and varied sexual fantasies; wanted sex more often; wanted a greater number of partners; liked a greater variety of sex acts; masturbated more frequently; showed deceased willingness to forego sex; showed more initiating and less refusing of sex; and were willing to take risks and incur more costs for sex. The authors noted: "We did not find a single study on any of nearly a dozen different measures that found women had a stronger sex drive than men. We think that the combined quantity, quality, diversity and convergence of the evidence render the conclusion [that men have stronger sex drives] indisputable (Baumeister et al., 2001)."

Masturbation is considered by sex researchers to be one of the purest measures of sex drive because it is not constrained as much by external factors (e.g. by having a partner or the risk of pregnancy or disease) than partnered sex, and in most studies men show higher levels of masturbation than women. For example in a British survey 73% of men and 36.8% of women reported masturbating in the previous four weeks (Gerressu et al., 2007). An American survey showed that in the age group of twenty-five to twenty-nine-year-olds, 5% of women and 20.1% of men reported masturbating more than four times a week. The gap closed somewhat when the frequency was reduced to multiple times per month with 21.5% of women and 25.4% of men in the twenty-five- to twenty-nine-year-old age group endorsing this frequency. However, the gender disparity remained throughout all age groups, with women being 10–15% lower than men in each category (Herbenick, 2010).

'I discovered self-pleasuring at about age twelve, and I've jacked off nearly every day, sometimes two or three times, for the past half-century. I don't spend nearly as much time on each wanking session as I did early on. As a teenager, I could go on and on for an hour or more before I allowed myself to spew. I don't have the patience for that anymore, so I usually yank one off in just a few minutes. I've done it everywhere – standing outside, sitting at my desk at work, walking with my hand in my pants pocket, and whilst driving a car.' – **Gus**

Similarly, we've all heard of the myth that men think about sex every seven seconds … and research shows that men *do* think about sex more frequently (the median being nineteen times a day) than women (the median being ten times a day). However, the researchers noted that there is a lot of variability amongst people. They also made a point of noting that typical men will think about sex statistically no more or less than they think about eating and sleeping. Also, researchers noted that the more comfortable someone was with his or her sexuality, the more likely they were to think about sex (Fisher et al., 2012).

It is this "comfort" with our sexuality that may be seen to confound the data around gender differences in desire more broadly. Our experience of desire is not only affected by our biology but also by our culturally learnt ease around sex. For example, one study found that men accepted an invitation for casual sex much more readily than women when they were approached at a nightclub or at a college campus. However, this gender difference disappeared when women were instead shown pictures of potential casual sex partners. The researchers attribute the difference to women feeling safer in this later circumstance (Baranowski & Hecht, 2015).

'I have always wanted sex more than the men I was in relationships with. I can't say that I'm "normal" or "abnormal" in that. But I am a woman and that is my experience. Many women would not admit to the above. Women are socialised to believe that they are supposed to want sex less and have more obstacles to enjoying sex. Women have been taught to fear sex. Physical, social, emotional and moral consequences are all attached to female sexuality.

'Given all these pressures and conditions placed on female sexuality, it makes sense that a woman's natural sex drive is heavily hampered, and if somehow she escapes this conditioning, she will usually lie to save face.' – **Jasmine**

MEN DON'T *JUST* WANT SEX

Biologically, men and women may actually be more similar than our sexpectations would have us believe in regards to desire and sex drive. Brain scans have shown that what happens in women's brains is pretty much the same as what happens in men's brains when they look at sexual imagery (Mitricheva, 2019). Testosterone – the sex hormone most often associated with sex drive – is commonly thought to account for the difference in sex drive between men and women (and also the variation between different men and women). However, research has shown no link between testosterone and desire in men, instead suggesting that higher frequency of masturbation causes higher desire rather than testosterone (Anders, 2012). Similarly, other research has supported this in that, in both men and women, sexual activity influences testosterone rather than testosterone influencing sexual activity (Dabbs & Mohammed, 1992).

Although there are many theories of sexual desire, we can assume that biological, social and personal or relational factors all play a part in a person's experience of sexual desire (Levine, 1987). Additionally, both men and women seem to draw on gender stereotypes to develop their sexpectations and construct their sexual experiences in a variety of aspects of sex, including around desire. It is entirely possible that many men experience higher sex drive than women because, in our society, we expect them to!

However, there are many men whose experiences are contrary to these gendered norms. For example, despite, and perhaps because of, this sexpectation, as many as 15% of men have "persistent complaints of low sexual desire" (Rosen, 2000). In heterosexual couples, men and women are equally likely to report having low sexual desire relative to their partner (Mark, 2012) and male and female libidos are equally influenced by things such as depression, stress levels and relationship satisfaction.

Both men and women have also been shown to draw on gender stereotypes to predict how much foreplay and intercourse their partners preferred, with women significantly underestimating men's desired length of foreplay (Miller & Byers, 2004). Similarly, stereotypes that suggest men are uninterested in kissing, cuddling and other forms of romance are not held up by research (e.g. Herbenick et al., 2017; Heiman et al., 2011).

When researching her book *Not Always in the Mood: The New Science of Men, Sex and Relationships* (2019), Sarah Hunter found that contrary to our outdated sexpectations, men wanted to feel desired by their partners and be told they were sexy; men wanted to feel emotionally connected during sex; men reported faking desire and having sex in order to please their partners; they reported enjoying an egalitarian approach to sex rather than always feeling they had to be the initiator; and they said that their desire was more fragile and susceptible to outside influences including lack of sleep, sickness and stress.

> *'The myth is that men are a sex toy that you can pull out of your closet and we're always ready to go when you are … Well, no, that's not actually the case. If your time and energy is spent on the adulting – paying bills, working overtime, trying to keep your energy up for elderly parents or young kids – is there really time to connect emotionally and build that bridge that ends up in the bedroom?'* – **Chris**

Gender and culture affect science, and science influences our beliefs about the world. In the area of sexuality, many scientists saw promiscuity in males and coyness in females in the animal kingdom because it fit their culturally endorsed sexpectations. It was a vicious cycle where sexpectations led the research, and then the research was used as evidence to back the sexpectations. New technology such as molecular paternity analysis has disproven these assumptions, and it has been found that across the animal kingdom, females frequently mate with multiple males and produce broods with multiple fathers. In the book *Promiscuity: An Evolutionary History of Sperm Competition,* it was concluded that "generations of reproduction biologists assumed females to be sexually monogamous but now it is clear that is wrong" (Birkhead, 2000). In the same line, when we look at the sexpectations in our own species, we find plenty of evidence that some traditional and scientifically endorsed ideas about sex are less natural than we thought.

For example, one argument that has been used against homosexuality is that it is unnatural because animals don't practise it. However, in populations of Japanese macaques, fruit flies, flour beetles, albatrosses, bottlenose dolphins and more than 500 other species, homosexual behaviour has been observed (Hogenboom, 2015). Similarly, the idea of the insatiable, horny "animal" homo sapien male and the demure, relationship-oriented female, may influence both women and men's construction of their own sexuality but does not necessarily represent a natural "truth".

GRINDIN' GAYS AND LESBIAN BED DEATH BY JAMES

Even in the same-sex world, the stereotypes of gay men always being DTF (down to fuck) and lesbians ending up in sexless relationships perpetuate gendered sexpectations.

Traditionally, gay men have been positioned as promiscuous. The gay male sex drive was the force behind Grindr, the original queer dating app. This app helped pioneer geo-social-based dating apps and modern dating as we know it when it launched in 2009. Gay men were responsible for the first sex-on-premises bath houses. Gay men have also been stereotypically more open to non-monogamous sexual relationships.

Queer culture, in general, has fought against heteronormativity and, for some, throwing out monogamy is an important part of rejecting heteronormative constructs and maintaining an image of being "sexually progressive". Having said that, not all same-sex attracted people identify as queer, and many don't have an issue wanting to lead a heteronormative life – picture a married couple, white picket fence, two kids and a dog, etc.

However, for those of us who grew up in the noughties and earlier, it was very difficult to even imagine that that could happen. We had little to no support in having same-sex partners whilst we were growing up, and many of us were encouraged to pursue heterosexual relationships. Marriage equality was a fantasy, many couples felt uncomfortable holding hands in the street, and it was next to impossible to have children. Perhaps the reason gay men have been stereotyped as "promiscuous" is because that was the only socially sanctioned option for us until recently?

In contrast, there is a stereotype that when two women are in a relationship with each other the passion dies off quickly. They become more like roommates than lovers. The term for this – "lesbian bed death" – was coined following research finding that lesbians have less sex than any other couples. Approximately half of lesbians in long-term (two years or longer) relationships reported that they had sex once a month or less (Blumstein & Schwartz, 1983).

A majority of comparative studies in the past thirty years have replicated these results, although a few have found no differences between lesbian and heterosexual couples. However, perhaps "sexual frequency" is not the best measure to assess lesbian sex by, particularly when there is no common standard with which to measure what constitutes a sexual encounter when there is no penis? Rather, lesbians report more frequent orgasms, longer lovemaking, and equivalent sexual satisfaction to their heterosexual counterparts (Blair & Pukall, 2014) – so, not quite as dead in bed as we have been led to believe!

Being same-sex oriented can allow us to explore different aspects of our sex lives and relationships without the traditions that heteronormative society dictates. We might find it even easier to make our own rules and walk our own path than our heterosexual counterparts, whether it comes to sexual frequency or some other sexpectation. What really matters is that we're honest with ourselves with what we really want, rather than following a script provided to us by either the generation before us, or the people around us.

EXERCISE: HOW HORNY ARE YOU REALLY?

When do you remember first experiencing sexual desire? Have you had periods of life since then when your desire has been higher or lower? What do you attribute that to?

How did you learn that your sex drive was normal or abnormal?

Have you ever had a partner who has a sex drive that disrupted your sexpectations (e.g. a woman with a higher sex drive than you if you are a man or a man who has refused sex)? How did you interpret that? Did it cause any concerns in your relationship?

How often would you like to have sex ideally? Does this match with how often you currently masturbate? If there is a difference, why do you think this is?

Have you ever noticed a link between your masturbation frequency and your sex drive?

CHAPTER 10

THE PRIMACY OF PENETRATION

LOSING OUR V-CARD

In human culture, "having sex" is still synonymous with penetration, specifically PIV (Penis in Vagina) in the heterosexual community. Although we have come a long way from sex being permitted purely for procreation, the act that is most associated with making babies is still given the starring role when it comes to sex.

Many people who are not bound by religious prohibitions have sex before marriage and, as such, the sexpectation of "saving yourself until marriage" is no longer a dominant one. Most statistics put the average age of loss of virginity between 16.8 years and 17.5 years, and these ages have been relatively stable across the last few decades, across English-speaking Western cultures (e.g. the USA, UK & Australia) and with little gender difference (Wellings et al., 2006).

However, few of you will be surprised when I specify that "loss of virginity" refers to age of first PIV intercourse. So, PIV can be seen as fundamental to our very first ideas of what "sex" involves (Laumann et al., 2004). It is the "home base" that teenagers aspire to reach and is a necessary act to lose one's "V-card".

> *'I lost my virginity during my first year of college when I was eighteen. Initially, he had a hard time inserting his penis into my vagina because my vagina was tight from never having had a penis inside it. But after a lot of pushing and squirming, he managed. My vagina was in a world of pain. The sex was tentative, uncomfortable, and lasted a few minutes (a few minutes too long, in my opinion). It hurt a lot (though I didn't bleed), but I told myself not to tell him to stop until he had orgasmed because I wanted the complete penetration-to-ejaculation experience.'* – **Janet**

The primacy of PIV as the "loss of virginity" is an old and enduring sexpectation. The controversial 1975 book *Forever* by Judy Blume was banned in many American high schools because of its detailed depiction of its protagonist Katherine losing her virginity to "Ralph", her boyfriend's penis. Notably for our discussion, the couple are frustrated in their first attempt to "have sex" (i.e. achieve PIV) as Katherine had her period. In 2007, a content analysis of *Seventeen* magazine's sex and health advice columns between 1982 and 2001 showed PIV as the defining act of virginity loss and, in turn, what it means to have had "real" sex. *Seventeen* classified oral sex and digital penetration as sexual "acts" as opposed to "sex", privileging the male penis as a necessary component for sex to occur (Medley-Rath, 2007).

Of course, these statistics are based on a heteronormative definition of virginity. And when you solely define the loss of virginity in terms of whether a penis has penetrated a vagina, you leave little room for those who don't want to have male/female penetrative sex to describe or validate their experiences. In fact, it could be said that the heteronormative assumption that women and men are "made for each other" is perpetuated through the common definition of *"the* sex act" as vaginal penetration by the penis (Jackson, 2006).

GAY VIRGINS
(By James)

Before I lost my "virginity", I remember thinking, *If I'm penetrated, does that mean I lose my bottoming virginity? What happens if I top? Is that a different type of virginity?* and, *How does this work for lesbians?!*

Unsurprisingly very little research has been done into how same-sex-attracted people view virginity and what it means to lose it. One study found that more gay men thought receiving anal intercourse (bottoming) was the definition of losing one's virginity, rather than being the penetrative partner (topping) (Huang, 2018).

The significance of being penetrated may be because of the perceived power imbalance. Being penetrated is a vulnerable act, which is perhaps why losing one's virginity is tied up with the act of penetration. However, there is also a power that comes with bottoming. I believe Samantha Jones from TV series *Sex and the City* put it best when she said, 'Maybe you're on your knees, but you got him by the balls.' Then there is the "power bottom" – a more active, receptive partner. So, being receptive doesn't have to mean being powerless.

There is even less research available on what constitutes losing your virginity when you're a same-sex-attracted woman. Those unfamiliar with lesbian sex can wonder if sex between women is even considered "sex" if there is no penetration. Notably one study found that most people they studied associated lesbian sex with vaginal penetration by a phallic substitute, such as a dildo (Pham, 2016). Thankfully, a woman into women would correct us pretty quickly – there need not be penetration for sex to occur!

'In terms of how society defines heterosexual sex as intercourse between a man and a woman, I feel like if I had to give a standard definition, it would be a million times easier to say well gay men have anal sex, but no one really knows what lesbians do, ever. I mean, I've had people just ask me, "Well, how do you have sex?" Like, well … what day of the week is it? I feel like it's a lot less definable simply because society defines sex as penetration. So, because there's no natural penis in a same-sex female relationship, it's a lot less easy to define.' – **Dana**

Perhaps there is a lack of research around loss of virginity when same-sex attracted because the milestone itself is not as important to a same-sex-attracted person as the milestone of "coming out". If virginity is a social construction that came about because of the commodification of women and the need to ensure legitimate heirs, then it has comparatively little relevance to the LGBT+ community who do not practise heteronormative reproductive sex. The act of identifying oneself outside the heteronormative model in terms of identity and claiming one's sexual rights by "coming out" is far more meaningful.

PIV = SEX

Though definitions of what constitutes having sex have become broader over the past few decades, PIV is still seen as central to the sexual act (Gavey et al., 1999). For example, in one study, 59% of respondents said that oral–genital contact did not qualify as "having sex" (Sanders and Reinisch, 1999). Another study found that both vaginal and anal intercourse were considered sex by most respondents but whether oral intercourse was labelled as sex depended on gender and whether orgasm occurred (Bogart et al., 2000). In one study, asking about the participants' most recent sexual encounter, for most couples the erotic dance involved three actions: PIV occurring in almost 100% of couples, mutual genital–hand massage (75%) and oral sex (25%) (Richter et al., 2006).

Equating "sex" with PIV alone is often the cause of distress people feel when they are unable to achieve PIV sex, or feel they can't satisfy a partner with PIV. In my experience it is issues like having a small penis, erectile dysfunction and vaginismus or vaginal pain that leads many hetero couples and single individuals to sex therapy. Although lack of an erection does not stop many forms of satisfying sexual contact, many men will seek therapy or take a PDE5 inhibitor such as sildenafil (Viagra) to regain their ability to penetrate.

Such is our obsession with erections and penetration that since it was released in 1998, Viagra has been prescribed to more than sixty-four million men worldwide (Connelly, 2017). It has made Pfizer, the drug company that manufactures it, more than 1.4 billion US dollars a year and, it was so popular that the online counterfeit market and other off-patent competition caused the company to release a lower-cost version in 2017.

Although Viagra has been placed in the history books alongside the contraceptive pill for its role in reducing shame, opening up discussion and liberating sexuality, as Pfizer Marketing Executive Dorothy Wetzel said, Viagra allowed for a "kind of Peter Pan fantasy" where men could be "forever their essential vital selves" (quoted in MacNeill, 2018). Viagra and similar drugs have also been increasingly used as a performance enhancement drug – to improve sexual performance or to counter the use of other recreational drugs, and it has been suggested that many millennials take it because they watch a lot of pornography and feel pressure to perform like a porn star.

'The times when I've been unable to perform have been some of the most emasculating moments of my life. I felt frustrated, infuriated at myself: I hated my body. I wanted to please my partner, but I had so little control. I worried that she felt unwanted or unsexy because of my ED. My partner thinks I take Viagra now and then, but I would be too embarrassed to tell her how often I actually take it – basically every time we have sex. But it's helped me feel better about myself. I would much rather take Viagra than an antidepressant.' – **Matt**

Under similar pressure to have PIV sex, many women with vaginismus (a condition where vaginal muscles spasm involuntarily and prevent penetration), sexual pain, or a similar issue that prevents penetration from occurring will feel sexually deficient. A significant proportion of women (7.5% in one British study (Mitchell et al., 2017)) experience varying levels of genital pain during sexual intercourse and experience significant personal and relationship distress.

'I was convinced that something was wrong with me. I was so ashamed — ashamed because on the one hand, I was having sex and felt uncomfortable telling doctors or therapists about it. And on the other hand, I was ashamed because I couldn't do "it", not all the way, not without it feeling like someone was stabbing my vagina with fifty different-sized knives.' – **Nina**

The emphasis on PIV sex for women is also out of proportion to the necessity of it for sexual pleasure. Although pornos would have you believe differently, most women report that it is easier to achieve orgasm through clitoral stimulation and comparatively few report that they can achieve orgasm through PIV alone. For example, in one of the largest surveys of sexual activity ever conducted, 50% of women experienced orgasm through PIV alone and 86% when their last sexual encounter involved manual stimulation and oral sex. This study found that the single largest predictor of a woman reaching orgasm during their last PIV intercourse was the number of activities other than PIV that the couple had engaged in immediately prior to PIV (Richters et al., 2006).

Similarly, a large American survey revealed that although both men and women rated vaginal penetration appealing, far more pleasing were those behaviours commonly associated with romance and affection. Saying sweet, romantic things during sex; kissing more often during sex; cuddling more often; and setting up the room to feel more romantic were all deemed more attractive than PIV (Herbenick et al., 2017.) In fact, many researchers have found a significant and strong relationship between affectionate behaviours and sexual satisfaction.

PENETRATION AND GAYS
(By James)

Some say that the straight world could learn a lot from the gay world, and around this sexpectation of penetration, I agree! PIA (penis in anus) is just one of many acts that are generally discussed between two gay men before they agree to hook up. It is not a taken-for-granted expectation, but must be explicitly agreed upon. Just because we have a prostate, doesn't mean we all like anal!

There are many reasons for this. Some guys like to douche before PIA and therefore a certain amount of planning and preparation needs to happen. There is also more acceptance of the idea that not all guys are into all things (e.g. some like to top, some like to bottom, others are versatile). Therefore, like in the kink world, we take greater care checking that our sexual turn-ons match up with our partners and don't just assume they will. Finally, I'd like to think that with the amount of sex most gays stereotypically have, we've worked out what we like and what we don't, and are more comfortable talking about it.

PIV AND "CHEATING"

The primacy of penetrative sex, and specifically PIV, in the heterosexual world has implications for notions of sexual fidelity. Is it considered "cheating" if you haven't had PIV sex?

One study asked participants to rate cheating on a scale of 0 to 100 (where 100 was definitely cheating): PIV scored 97.7, oral sex 96.8, kissing on the lips 88.7, erotic texts 82.6, hand holding 63.2, and forming a deep emotional bond 52.4 (Kruger et al., 2013). Additionally, some studies report that men and women have different views on what they consider cheating, with men more threatened by and less likely to forgive physical cheating than emotional infidelity (e.g. Bendixen et al., 2018).

In line with this gender difference, many couples exploring non-monogamy will begin with rules such as a "one-penis policy" – where a woman is only allowed to have "one penis" in her romantic and sexual life but often sexual exploration with other women is allowed. Dating back to early polygynous cultures, and legitimacy and succession concerns, this boundary helps protect the couple from male sexual jealousy as they explore opening up their relationship.

In reality, the process of infidelity (and most processes of consensual opening up) is gradual and can be a slippery slope. No one just all of a sudden, accidentally ends up with their P in a V (or V around a P for that matter!). However, the sexpectation that PIV sex is the only "real" sex allows some people to deny the importance of emotional or physical behaviour that their partners may consider unfaithful or in violation of their boundaries, because it's not "sex".

'I know even though cheating is still cheating, there are varying degrees of cheating and some forms are more intimate and hurtful than others. For instance, a one-night stand wouldn't be the same as an entire affair involving deep emotions.' – **Troy**

EXERCISE: A PARALLEL UNIVERSE WITHOUT PENETRATION

Have you ever had *really* good sex that did not involve penetration? Imagine you wake up tomorrow and you are in a parallel universe, one where penetration was not possible, nor even thought of. In this universe, PIV (or PIA) is considered as ridiculous as someone trying to shove a penis in a nostril (no, please don't try that!).

What do you imagine would happen to your sex life? What things would you be your go-to sex acts? What things would you be tempted to try? … In fact, why imagine? For a month, try banning penetration from your sexual repertoire and see what you notice.

CHAPTER 11

IT'S ALL ABOUT THE BIG "O"

DID YOU CUM?

From "you would know it if you've had one" to being described as "fireworks", the rhetoric that elevates the orgasm and defines it as the pinnacle of the sexual experience is everywhere. Every sexual encounter in every Hollywood film, every trashy romance novel, and every porno ends in orgasm … so you could be forgiven for assuming that orgasm is the proper goal and logical conclusion of the sexual act. But why stop at one? With the ready availability of porn, there are multiple orgasms, cum shots and female ejaculation to aspire to!

> 'He pushes inside me and rolls his hips. I lift mine to meet him and I'm exploding, falling apart and flying at the same time, dropping through the earth's core as my body tries to cope with these sensations … It is like being prodded by a hot iron, though: I am burning up. I explode angrily, loudly, my body shaking from head to toe, glistening with sweat.' (Connelly, 2018)

Studies have found that orgasm is always positioned as "the peak", the desired outcome of the sexual act and that the sexual act itself is defined as a linear process that culminates in orgasm (Potts, 2000). Even though many studies have reported that women on the whole are relatively indifferent to orgasm being necessary for their own enjoyment, they do feel their orgasm is necessary for the satisfaction of their partners (Nicholson & Burr, 2003; Bancroft, Loftus and Long, 2003).

Men report orgasms in approximately 95% of heterosexual encounters, but for women, depending on the study, the figure ranges from only 50–70%. An estimated 10–15% of women have never had an orgasm and, as we discussed previously, many more find it easier to achieve orgasm through clitoral stimulation rather than the PIV shown in the movies. An analysis of thirty-three studies over eighty years suggests that only 25% of women orgasm consistently and 50% sometimes orgasm through PIV (Lloyd, 2006).

One in three men report having experienced premature ejaculation (Carson & Gunn, 2006). What classifies as "premature", however, is up for debate and even though the official definition is ejaculating within one minute of PIV (yes, the primacy of PIV is even seen in this definition!), most men will consider themselves premature if they ejaculate before they are ready to, or before their partners orgasm – a pretty high goal post given the statistics on female orgasm above!

'After a couple weeks of having sex, I asked one night, "How do I know when you're close to coming?" … She said, "I don't cum." I was pretty confused. I felt naïve, but I didn't realise that some girls just can't cum through penetrative sex . I felt really disappointed. Like we were only having sex to get me off.' – **Phil**

Many people also don't know that men can orgasm without ejaculation. This "dry orgasm" can occur for a variety of medical reasons (such as after surgery to the bladder or prostate, or chemotherapy) but can also be trained with masturbation, Kegel (aka pelvic floor) exercises and a practice called "edging". The Taoists and Tantrikas used this technique for spiritual purposes but most men who practise it today do so because there is no refractory period (i.e. they can keep their erection after orgasm) and they can train their orgasm to last ten or more minutes.

Men can also ejaculate without orgasm, which is known as "ejaculatory anhedonia" or "anorgasmic ejaculation". This is also often because of medical reasons, vitamin or hormone imbalances. It is no surprise that no man really practises this one! Therefore, despite us only really seeing the classical orgasm and ejaculation "climax" scenario on movies and in pornos, a multitude of orgasm experiences are available to men. As Bernie Zilbergeld, author of *The New Male Sexuality* (1999), says: "sometimes there is no peak feeling and sometimes that feeling comes long before ejaculation. Some men don't have a lot of feeling when they ejaculate, and some men have lots of peak feelings, with and without ejaculations. There is no good and bad, right and wrong, about any of this".

At thirty-eight, I found my ejaculatory orgasms were getting weaker and weaker, as was my sexual potency (libido and erection strength). I was ejaculating daily and clearly this was no longer sustainable. By the end, I was experiencing non-orgasmic ejaculations. I remember feeling that my final "peak orgasm" was no more pleasurable than peeing when you've been needing to go for a while – hardly climactic.

'In desperation, I was searching online for solutions when I heard of the concept of non-ejaculatory orgasms – mini orgasms. Eventually through practice and building my pelvic-floor muscle group up, I was able to stop myself from ejaculating.

'Sometimes I can go up to a whole month without ejaculating yet experiencing the mini orgasms on a daily (or almost daily) basis. Other times the pressure build-up of going a month without ejaculating becomes too much and I just have to release. However, when I do ejaculate, no matter how much I try to relax and enjoy what most men refer to as "the happy ending", I just feel nothing or hardly anything at all.' – **Peter**

Women too can have different types of orgasm, although there is some disagreement amongst researchers on how to classify them. Most women report that "some orgasms are better than others" (Herbenick et al., 2017) and in non-academic articles, female orgasms have been divided into as many as four to fifteen types. For example, the "clitoral orgasm", which is produced by stimulation of the clitoris and clitoral bulbs is described as the fastest way for women to orgasm. Women describe experiencing them as a surge of pleasure originating from the clitoris – tingly, light and fun with a definitive build, a climax with pelvic contractions and then a feeling of descent.

The "G-spot orgasm" comes from stimulating the anterior wall of the vagina approximately one to two inches inside. These orgasms often require a longer period of stimulation (ten to thirty minutes) and feel more like waves of pleasure that spread throughout the body, starting from inside of the vagina. Similarly, the "cervical orgasm" is produced through stimulation of the cervix, and is described as extended, full-body waves of pleasure accompanied by a sense of peace and joy.

'Clitoral or contractive orgasms have a tense, high-pitched, build-up kind of feel to them. All this attention goes to one spot, such as my clit, and amps up and up and up, until I have a feeling of surrender and then the pleasurable sensitivity spreads to other parts of my body beyond that small genital area that's being stimulated.

'When I first experienced an expansive cervical orgasm, which was not very long ago, it was life-altering. This was more than the contractive sensations. A lot of what I was doing was gently massaging my deep vaginal walls and my cervix. The pleasure was slow in coming, and then, bit by bit, it became more pleasurable, exotic, a really loving sensation. I had this feeling of totally relinquishing my body to the experience ... Eventually I entered a kind of buzzed state, a period of plateau, in which not only did my entire body feel pleasurably, sensitively warm, but my mental state was calm, cool, colourful.' – **Jenny**

Female ejaculation, or "squirting", is one of the more well known and idealised forms of female orgasm because of its fetishisation in porn. Anything from a small amount to a cup's worth of fluid can be released from the urethra during orgasm after twenty-five to sixty minutes of sexual stimulation. Following controversy about what female ejaculate was, researchers tested the ejaculate of seven women. They confirmed that squirting is essentially the involuntary emission of urine from the bladder during sexual activity. However, in some of the women's squirt, there was some PSA (prostate-specific antigen), which is produced by the Skene glands, the female counterpart to the prostate (Salama et al., 2014). The women studied had emptied their bladders before beginning sexual stimulation. However, another ultrasound taken just before orgasm revealed that for unknown reasons their bladders completely refilled (imagine being a participant in that study!). This suggests that the ejaculation was indeed a sexual response and not an "accident".

What about for people who are not in the gendered bodies assigned to them at birth? It is a common misconception that transgender people are unable to orgasm after gender reassignment surgery. Studies have found that as many as 85% of transgender men and 100% of transgender women were able to orgasm (De Cuypere et al., 2005). The majority of the people studied reported a change in orgasmic feeling; towards more powerful and shorter for female-to-males, and more intense, smoother, and longer in male-to-females. Similarly, in a study of male-to-female transgender women, 82% reported that they could climax after surgery and 56% reported that their orgasms were more intense (Hess, 2014).

BLUE BALLS AND ORGASMIC HEALTH

In discourse dating back to medieval times, the orgasm has been awarded with various medical and mental health benefits. Many men assume that ejaculation at regular intervals is necessary for sexual health and the less sophisticated of those will use this argument as a way of influencing a partner to not be a "cock-tease", to have sex or to continue engaging in sex until they can ejaculate.

"Blue balls" – the name given to the experience of stopping sexual activity before ejaculation – is also known as epididymal hypertension (EH). It is the experience of aching in the testicles after having an erection without an orgasm and is sometimes accompanied by a blue-ish colour to the testicles from the build-up of blood in the veins. It is not common, it is not dangerous, and it is not just the prerogative of those with male genitals! People with female genitals can also experience vasocongestion and "blue vulva". Blue balls can be relieved through ejaculation (be it through partnered sex or solo masturbation), but also through simple distraction until the arousal has subsided.

Beyond blue balls, there have been many studies that have found that frequency of ejaculation and orgasm is protective of health in various ways. If you thought that we were fixated on achieving orgasm just because it felt good, think again! The hormones orgasm releases are suggested to have benefits for longevity, cancer risk, heart disease risk and immune function.

Once again, there are a lot of problems with the science in this area. Longitudinal studies can only make associations and cannot say for sure orgasm *causes* one or another health benefit, nor can they rule out all other factors. Similarly, just because certain hormones or antibodies are released with orgasm does not necessarily mean orgasm definitely produces positive health effects or that those hormones and antibodies couldn't also be produced in other ways. However, with that disclaimer out of the way, let's look at what the studies have shown.

Longevity has been linked to the frequency of orgasm for men and women in longitudinal studies. For example, in one well-reported study in Caerphilly, South Wales, 918 men aged 45–59 were given a physical examination, including a medical history, and blood pressure, electrocardiogram, and cholesterol screenings. They were also asked about their frequency of orgasm. At the ten-year follow-up, it was found that the mortality risk was 50% lower amongst men who had frequent orgasms (defined in this study as two or more per week) than amongst men who had orgasms less than once a month. Even when controlling for other factors such as age, social class and smoking status, the findings held out (Davey Smith et al.,

1997). Similarly, an analysis of 252 racially diverse people in North Carolina from 1941 over twenty-five years revealed that the predictors of longevity were frequency of intercourse for men, and past enjoyment of intercourse and higher frequency of orgasm for women (Friedman & Martin, 2011).

The idea that more frequent ejaculation can reduce the risk of prostate cancer has mixed evidence. Some studies say it does (e.g. Rider, 2016), some studies say it doesn't. One such study concluded that there was no protective relationship between ejaculation frequency and prostate cancer for most except those in the highest category (greater than twenty-one ejaculations per month) and in the lowest category (less than three ejaculations a month) (Leitzmann et al., 2004). Similarly, another study found that higher frequency (greater than five times a week) in early adult life (twenties) led to reduced risk (Giles et al., 2003). However, in opposition, masturbation more than once weekly in the twenties and thirties (not sex, just masturbation) was found to increase the risk of prostate cancer and, any sexual activity in the fifties reduced the risk (Dimitropoulou et al., 2009).

Low frequency of sexual activity (once a month) has been found to be associated with an increased risk of heart disease. Men who had sex at least twice a week were 50% less likely than their once-a-month peers to have a heart attack (Hall, et al., 2010). In the Caerphilly study mentioned above, men who reported low frequency of orgasms (less than once per month) also had rates of fatal heart attacks twice that of those who had reported high frequency of orgasms. It is thought that the steroid dehydroepiandrosterone (DHEA), which is released during orgasm, is responsible for this reduced risk – the assumption being that it is not the sex per se but the orgasm that is protective (Feldman et al., 1998).

Similarly, more sex (though not orgasm specifically) has been linked to a better immune system. One study showed that people who had sex once or twice a week had 30% higher levels of the antibody that helps stave off sickness, immunoglobulin A (IgA), than those who were abstinent. Interestingly, people who had sex more often than once or twice a week had IgA levels similar to those of abstainers (Charnetski & Brennan, 2004). Another study had eleven men masturbate until orgasm and drew their blood for analysis continuously throughout the process. (Who volunteers for these things?! No wonder they only got eleven!) They found that components of the immune system, the number of "killer cells" called leukocytes, were increased by both sexual arousal and orgasm (Haake et al., 2004).

Several hormones including oxytocin, endorphins, prolactin, vasopressin, DHEA, serotonin and dopamine are released during or after orgasm and all are lauded to have positive health effects. There are plenty of claims both academic and popular that orgasms can relieve stress and help you relax, help you sleep more soundly, can reduce pain, relieve migraines and improve your complexion. And that's in addition to the emotional effects of helping you feel close and connected, warm and satiated.

FAKING IT

But what about if you struggle to orgasm? Or if your orgasm isn't like you see in the pornos or movies? What about if the effort and pressure to reach orgasm means that you lose pleasure in the rest of your sexual experience? Many heterosexual men focus almost exclusively on getting their partners to come to orgasm and withholding their own orgasm before this is achieved. Many heterosexual women feel great pressure to reach orgasm to save their partner's feelings.

As a consequence, both men and women will "fake" orgasm rather than make non-orgasmic sex a permissible and enjoyable part of their sexual repertoire. A random-sample telephone poll of 1,501 Americans showed that 48% of women and 11% of men faked orgasm, usually to please their partner or "get it done" (Langer et al., 2004). For anyone who has ever experienced this, questioning the sexpectation that good sex is all about the "big O" could be a game changer.

'I've faked only a few times with my current girlfriend whilst I was recovering from a basketball-related groin injury. As soon as I faked it, she said, "Did you really?" and I had to escape to the bathroom, close the door, and dispose of the evidence — or lack of it. After a few more fakes, she called me on it. She said, "You're not coming. Don't lie to me." She says that I make a very specific face, and I wasn't doing it right.' – **Tim**

'I'm a woman who fakes orgasms a decent amount — about once every five to six times. I wouldn't consider it a problem really — it's not like I feel like I'm not fulfilled sexually. I still enjoy having sex with my husband, even if it's not always orgasmic. Unfortunately, he thinks that my orgasm — not once, or twice, but three times — is absolutely necessary and without it, sex doesn't count. Sometimes faking an orgasm actually gets me more turned on, sometimes it's just not going to work and my vag becomes sore and dry. Sometimes I do orgasm, but it's very quiet. So I re-do it more vocally so I let him know, audibly, that he's doing an excellent job.' – **Tilly**

EXERCISE: ORGASM OR CHOREGASM?

Have you experienced different types of orgasm? Did you prefer a particular type?

How important is orgasm to you? Why do you think it is important?

Do you ever fake orgasm? What feelings and thoughts would you have if you talked to your partner about not making orgasm the goal instead?

Have you ever made the mistake of assuming your partner wanted to orgasm? How did you find out it was a mistake?

How would you end a sexual encounter if you and your partner agreed that orgasm would not be the end point?

CHAPTER 12

SEXPERTS

THE PORNIFICATION OF SEX

In recent years, attitudes have shifted and our culture has never been more tolerant of sex in almost every way. Most people now think that sex between unmarried adults and same-sex sex is "not wrong at all" (e.g. Twenge et al., 2015) and polyamory is close to being a household word. Sex has fewer consequences than it did in previous generations, in the Western world contraction of HIV is now much less common and most women can access birth control easily.

Accessing sex and sexual material is far easier: casual sex apps make obtaining sex easy; graphic sex scenes are portrayed on prime-time TV; song lyrics and music clips contain increasingly erotic content. Mainstream television and film, such as *Sex in the City* and *Fifty Shades of Grey* have changed how we feel about sex toys and have turned what used to be shamefully called "perversion" into exciting "kink". Vibrators have become just another bedroom accessory and BDSM has been transformed into "mummy porn" – porn tame enough that it is accessible to the suburban "soccer mom"

(Lierberman, 2017). Even the taboo on anal sex has lifted – anal "fifth base" has become so mainstream that *Teen Vogue* ran a guide to it (Engle, 2019)!

The media has become an influential source of – albeit often inaccurate – sex education (Kunkel et al., 2005). Studies have shown that the sexual content viewed in the media influences adolescent sexual behaviour and that media have at least as great an influence on sexual behaviour and their sexpectations as religion or a young person's relationship with their parents and peers (e.g. Collins et al., 2011).

If that's just general media, what about porn?

Porn of all kinds is free and available on our smartphone in case our bus trip gets boring. Indeed, in the latest data released from Pornhub, 2018 saw 80% of their traffic coming from smartphones and tablets.

Numbers of people and frequency of porn viewing is continually rising whilst the average age of first viewing is lowering. Recent statistics have put the average age of first exposure to porn at thirteen years old, with 44% of that being accidental. These same authors found a link between how first exposure to porn at a younger age leant towards the greater valuing of power over women (Bischmann et al., 2017).

'I saw my first porn when I was eight years old – I was sort of shocked by it, but fascinated as well. It just seemed so real. I'd never really seen people naked before and here they were, naked and doing things to each other … By the time I was fourteen watching porn had become my favourite thing to do. I was constantly searching for something new on the internet that would give me a bigger high. I gave up playing footy and stopped seeing my mates so I could stay up all night watching porn instead. To make it feel more real, I would seek out women on chatrooms to act out

scenarios. I used to ask girls to do things and get off on that, rather than enjoying the pleasure of sex. Eventually I couldn't get aroused by girls anymore.' – **Adam**

The maxim "if it exists, there is porn of it" is absolutely true! In 2018, Pornhub reported that its daily visits exceeded one hundred million (for perspective, that's the equivalent of the combined populations of Canada, Poland and Australia visiting every day!). To satisfy this audience, Pornhub's amateurs, models and content partners uploaded an incredible 4.79 million new videos that year, creating over 1 million hours of new content to watch on the site – that's 115 years' worth of viewing!

Because of our high-speed internet streaming, the amount of porn we can watch exponentially outpaces the amount of sex we have. We also have access to more extreme porn than the sex most of us will ever have – or potentially even want – in our own lives. For some, particularly the younger generation, porn is just one more digital activity that they use to relieve stress or create a diversion, much like social media and binge watching TV. However, there are conflicting opinions as to the extent to which people see their porn life and their sex life as entirely separate things.

As discussed earlier, decades of research on the effects of pornography has shown that porn usage influences people's (especially young people's) expectations about sex and shapes their sexual practices (Heldman & Wade, 2010). For example, anal intercourse, facial ejaculation, sex with multiple partners and deep fellatio sexual acts have all increased because of their prevalence in mainstream hetero porn (Quadara et al., 2017).

But whilst these more permissive attitudes about sex and sexual practices themselves may not be inherently problematic, the most dominant, popular and accessible porn contains messages and behaviours about sex, gender, power and pleasure that are *very* problematic. In particular, the rise of unsafe sex without condoms and sexual violence has also been linked to porn usage and many straight women report a proclivity for new hook-up partners to "choke" them or "slap" their vulva (without first obtaining consent) during sex. This physical aggression (slapping, choking, gagging, hair pulling) and verbal aggression such as name-calling is predominantly portrayed as done by men to their female partners in hetero porn.

More and more we are becoming porn-literate, porn-saturated and our own at-home porn stars. We see porn, and in a never-ending feedback loop, we each have the ability to replicate, reinvent, share and upload. And so we reach the chicken-or-egg question: do we have sex this way because of porn, or does porn look like this because this is how we like to have sex – or would like to have sex if our bodies were that firm, our genitalia that responsive and we had all the requisite toys?

The Kinsey Reports of the 1950s were the first comprehensive attempts to document how men and women participated in various sexual activities. It could be said that Pornhub is the Kinsey Report of the modern day, journalling the huge range of erotic desires and sexual behaviours we are now exposed to and participate in.

BARBIE-BODIED AND PRESSURED TO PERFORM

We live in a world flooded by the idealised notions of perfect bodies, adventurous sex and proficient partners. Women and men are expected to be knowledgeable about sex, enjoy sex and engage relatively regularly in a variety of sexual practices. As such, when our real-life sex doesn't turn out like this, it's easy for us to think that something is wrong.

We all go into our sexual experiences with an idealised movie (often a porno!) in our heads of what we should look like, how we should sound, how many positions we should cover and what sex acts we should be up for. We also have idealised sexpectations about how our bodies should perform. We can get so caught up in performing this movie that we lose contact with our actual bodily experience – a certain pathway to sexual performance problems! Compared to previous generations, we may be "sexperts" but our expertise is in what society is telling us we *should* want, and most of us have very little expertise in discovering and communicating what we *actually* want.

Discovering your sexual preferences takes time under the best of circumstances, and our current context of hooking up and pornification does not encourage this. Research suggests that, for most people, and particularly for women, sex with a regular partner tends to be better than casual sex (Pederson and Blekesaune, 2003; Richters et al., 2006; Waite & Joyner, 2001). It is proposed that this is because of the learning of "partner-specific sexual skills" – i.e. knowing what your partner likes and how their body responds. As one author notes, "sex with the partner who knows what one likes and how to provide it is bound to be more satisfying than sex with a partner who lacks such skills" (Waite & Joyner, 2001). It is also potentially due to the increased emotional satisfaction, comfort and sexual freedom within the context of a longer sexual relationship.

Modelling your behaviour after what you've seen on screen can lead to what is termed "spectatoring". Spectatoring is where you get stuck in your head, focusing from a third-person perspective on how you look, how you sound, or how you are performing rather than focusing on your bodily experience of sensation and pleasure or focusing on your partner. Spectatoring is well known to increase sexual-performance fears, sexual dissatisfaction and negatively impact sexual functioning (Masters & Johnson, 1970). Indeed, many people feel pressured to emulate porn actors and actresses – to achieve orgasm from penetration alone, be rock-hard from the beginning and stay rock-hard throughout, to participate in thirty minutes or more of vigorous sex without ejaculation, to be vocal during sex, to make her orgasm multiple times with the flick of a finger or tongue, to squirt, etc.

> 'Adult actress here. I know people say they know this, but viewers really don't understand how long it takes to film a video and how fake it all is. I've been in over forty pornos, they're usually half an hour or so long for each scene. But I'm on set for anywhere from five to twelve hours … Also, don't be one of those idiots who expects your SO to do everything you see in a porno. If it looks like we're holding that crazy fucking position for five minutes, it's more like thirty-second clips – I'll ask for a cut, go smoke a cigarette, stretch, slap some lube on and get back in it.' – **Cindy**

Both male and female consumers of pornography report increased levels of self-objectification and body surveillance (Quadara et al., 2017). This results in general body self-consciousness, which has been shown to have a number of deleterious sexual effects. For example, body self-consciousness has been linked to decreased sexual pleasure, decreased ability to be aroused, poorer sexual functioning, poor sexual assertiveness and self-esteem as well as higher levels of sexual avoidance, and sexual risk-taking (Berman et al. 2003; Yamamiya et al., 2006; Mullinax et al., 2015).

In this way, for many people worries about how they look is one of the biggest things that impede them being present and enjoying sex. Our society has a very narrow range of what it considers attractive and sexy, and most people will deviate from that ideal in some way. As a result of this self-consciousness, many people will avoid sex, or limit their sex life to only having sex in certain positions or with low light to avoid revealing their body. Rather than question their sexpectations around what bodies are "sexy", they instead blame themselves for eating "too much" or not working out "enough".

Along with making us more self-conscious, sexpectations developed from porn viewing decrease our satisfaction with our own "real" bodies. Frequency of porn viewing is associated with increased concern about penis size in men (Cranney, 2015). Similarly, women requesting cosmetic genitoplasty or breast enlargement will often bring pornographic pictures of breasts and/or vulvae to their cosmetic surgeons to illustrate their desired appearance (Braun, 2005; Liao & Creighton, 2007).

It makes sense that general female-genital-appearance satisfaction, breast-size satisfaction and male-penis-size satisfaction make for better sex. And indeed, many studies have found that these positive body perceptions are associated with sexual confidence, satisfaction and frequency (Berman et al., 2003; Ålgars et al., 2011; Morrison, 2005).

Porn viewing also negatively impacts our perceptions of our partners' bodies. However, our decreased satisfaction does not stop at physical appearance. After consumption of porn, both genders reported less satisfaction with their intimate partners – with their physical appearance but also with these partners' affection, sexual curiosity and sexual performance (Zillmann & Bryant 1988; Weaver et al., 1984).

It has been proposed that the recent explosion of the "amateur" category of porn indicates that people are moving away from commercially produced porn and wanting to see more natural bodies. "Amateur" was Pornhub's third most popular category in 2018. So, watching improbably perfect bodies engaging in acrobatic acts in decadent settings may be becoming less exciting and many are beginning to prefer the low-fi realism of actors and actresses who could be the "girl/boy next door".

EXERCISE: DIY PORN STAR

Thinking about the porn you have seen, what would you like to try in your own sex life and what do you think you watch "just for the fun of it"? Why?

Have you yourself, or have you been with a partner who has been quite self-conscious during sex? What did it do for your experience?

How do you measure your own sexual performance? Where do you think you got those goal posts from?

What would be the greatest compliment someone could give you sexually? Why is this important to you?

Thinking back to your description of one of your best sexual experiences, which parts of it would fit in in a porno? Are there elements that wouldn't?

Do you think it's possible to be a "sexpert"? If so, is being a "sexpert" about knowing techniques or performing various acts or something else? Thinking back on your own experiences with a great lover, what was it about how they were sexually, that made the sex so great?

CHAPTER 13

THE MEANING OF SEX

BEYOND BABIES

Until relatively recent times, when asked "Why do people
have sex?" most answers would probably include a reference
to reproduction. Until the first "test-tube baby" in 1978,
sex was the only way babies could be made. Since then,
there have been an estimated eight million IVF (In Vitro
Fertilization) babies born (Scutti, 2018). The advances
in, and availability of, reliable contraception and rapid
developments in IVF reproductive technology have
effectively separated sex acts from procreation so that today,
most acts of PIV sex do not result in a live birth.

Because LGBT+ people have long been excluded from
traditionally accepted expressions of sex and love – the
biological procreative kind – they have by necessity been
trendsetters in forging their own sexual practices and
relationship norms. From "leather men" (the forefathers of
the current kink scene), sex-on-premises saunas, to the first
hook-up app technology, same-sex oriented people have
pioneered cultural groups, places and technology to enjoy sex

without meaning. They have also been seen to lead the way in acceptance of non-monogamous relationships. Recent analysis of data from the USA found that 32% of gay men, 5% of lesbians and 22% of bisexual-identified people reported being in open relationships compared to 4–5% of the general population (Levine et al., 2018).

In general, we now have more accepting attitudes towards premarital and same-sex activity. Where in the US in the early 1970s premarital sex was accepted by 29%, it rose to being accepted by 58% of people in the period between 2010 and 2012. Similarly, attitudes towards same-sex-oriented sex was accepted by less than 20% before 1993, but rose to 44% in 2012, and 56% for the generation born after 1982 (Twenge et al., 2015). The same attitudinal shift can be seen in Australian and British data.

Sex without meaning – i.e. sex being purely for pleasure, an end unto itself – can also be seen in the "hook-up" culture that has developed since the early noughties. Occurring on a college campus or through dating-app technology, a "hook-up" can include any form of physical sexual activity, usually without the expectation of emotional bonding or long-term commitment. Many authors argue that increased access to porn via the internet spurred hook-up culture because it challenged the idea that "good sex" takes place in a monogamous relationship (Heldman & Wade, 2010).

The casual sex encounters characterised by the hook-up have been seen as an adaptation to the busy and achievement-oriented life we lead and the cultural shift towards the delay of marriage and children in favour of career (Garcia et al., 2013). Hook-up culture has caused great outcry amongst conservative journalists and social commentators, the likes of which has not been seen since the introduction of the oral contraceptive pill. However, many believe the reported shift away from "dating" and the search for a monogamous committed relationship in favour of "hooking up" is overstated (Luff et al., 2016).

'Now, this guy, we had the exact same background, same tastes, same challenges. I was very cautious, I spoke to him for almost two months before meeting him, but when we met, sparks flew (at least for me). We went back to my place and had a great time. But he left immediately afterwards, saying he had work the next day (it was a weekend!). The next day he blocked me. I know that hooking up doesn't generally go anywhere, but I felt pathetic, hurt, and so, so stupid.' – **Amy**

'One guy I hooked up with three times, and he said, "I love you" every time. That was evocative. But for some weird reason, I didn't run out – I was like, you know what? I'll say it right back. It felt right as we were making out, clothes still fully on, and he would say it. But I said to myself, you know what? It's nice to have someone say "I love you" to me during sex. As much as I knew it was absolutely insane to say that, that is quite possibly the most polite thing you can say to anyone.' – **Sam**

'Hook-ups tend to be based on aesthetics and sexual chemistry alone. I had sex with a lot of women who were absolutely not my type (vastly different interests, beliefs, etc.) and it was purely about the physical. If a girl took an emotional shine to me it was a turn-off. I was basically substituting self-worth for sex and it worked in the short term. That's not to say there weren't girls who I had feelings for, but my trust issues meant that I stifled the feelings and kept them at arm's length.' – **Rick**

The hook-up culture can be seen to be the latest dish in the "meaningless" sex banquet that began with prostitution (aka the "world's oldest profession") and has continued with pornography and the commercial sex trade in all its forms. Some say that even the hook-up is not "meaningless" in that a majority of people who engage in hook-ups report that they would like it to develop into a romantic relationship, although a very small percentage of these people (6.5% in one study) expect this to actually happen (Garcia & Reiber, 2008).

The shift in attitudes towards the acceptance of sex without "meaning" is, paradoxically, quite a meaningful development in contemporary life. It represents the first successful attempt to make sex as a recreational activity equally available to women and men, and (ideally) free of shame and guilt for both genders.

DOES MEANINGLESSNESS TURN US OFF?

There are two conflicting stories about the effect of more permissive attitudes towards sex. On the one hand, current generations are supposed to be Tinder-swiping, fuck-buddying pansexuals – the most sexually experimental generation since the ancient Greeks. Yet study after study has found that millennials have less sex than previous generations. Despite the ready availability of the hook-up, there has been a decline in the frequency of sex across age groups. In the USA, adults had sex about nine times fewer on average in the 2010s than they did in the 1990s – a 14% decline in sexual frequency (Twenge et al., 2017). People in their early twenties are two-and-a-half times more likely to not be having sex than Boomers were in their early twenties – with 15% reporting being virgins compared to 6% of Boomers at the same age.

Upon analysis, this study concluded that, contrary to popular opinion, the decline wasn't linked to longer working hours or pornography use but was instead due to an increasing number of people without a steady partner and a decline in sex amongst those who were partnered.

Some authors have begun to define this as a "sexual counter-revolution". They theorise that the benefits of having meaningless sex do not outweigh the potential consequences of STDs, pregnancy, sexual assault and sexual harassment claims. One commentator writes: "whereas the 1960s saw a freeing up of attitudes towards sex, pushing at boundaries, this counter-swing is turning sexual freedom into sexual fear and nearly all sexual opportunities into a legalistic minefield" (Murray, 2017).

The preference for screen-based social interactions over real ones may also contribute to the sex drought. Young people are living with their parents for longer, video games and online subscriptions for television shows and movies such as Netflix are on the rise and the average young person spends seven and a half hours with media each day – ten hours and forty-five minutes if one accounts for multiple media used simultaneously (Rideout et al., 2010).

Why should young men and women risk rejection, STDs and the anxiety of having to meet up with someone when you can chat to girls and boys on social media and watch porn in the privacy of your own bedroom? Indeed, most studies have found that acceptance of and an increase in masturbation has occurred in recent generations (Kontula & Haavio-Mannila, 2003). The Relationships in America Project survey of 15,738 people found that from 1992 to 2014, the number of American men who reported masturbating in a given week doubled to 54%, and the number of women more than tripled to 26% (Gordon et al., 2014).

> 'The internet has made it so easy to gratify basic social and sexual needs that there's far less incentive to go out into the "meat world" and chase those things. This isn't to say that the internet can give you more satisfaction than sex or relationships, because it doesn't [but it can] supply you with just enough satisfaction to placate those imperatives … I think it's healthy to ask yourself: "If I didn't have any of this, would I be going out more? Would I be having sex more?" For a lot of people my age, I think the answer is probably yes.' – **Chris**

There is also an increase in people identifying as asexual – although the term means different things to different people, it is generally used to describe someone who doesn't experience sexual attraction. Perhaps the increase is artificial, the greater tolerance for non-normative sexual preferences in recent times allowing more asexual people to better understand themselves and come out. However, there is also speculation that the constant exposure to sexual images in magazines and on television may have turned some people off sex rather than fuelling their interest.

"MAKING LOVE"

> 'To be loved, then, is preferable to intercourse, according to the nature of erotic desire. Erotic desire, then, is more a desire for love than for intercourse. If it is most of all for that, that is also its end. Either intercourse, then, is not an end at all or it is for the sake of being loved.' (Aristotle, fourth century BCE)

For Aristotle, the real reason we have sex is because we want to love and be loved. In support of this, one study found that most women reported that love was necessary for maximum satisfaction in a sexual relationship and that love made sex physically more pleasurable because they felt less inhibited and more free to explore their sexuality (Montemurro, 2014).

Similarly, for both men and women, feelings of mutual affection may enhance sex, whether or not it is accompanied by a long-term commitment. Studies have found that both sexes report greater emotional satisfaction in sexually exclusive relationships that they expect to last a long time (Waite & Joyner, 2001), whilst others have found that relationship satisfaction influences sexual satisfaction and vice versa (Christopher & Sprecher, 2000; Parish et al., 2007).

The importance of some form of relational intimacy for "good sex" has been shown to be important through reports from sex workers, who describe how many of their clients want to pretend that the sex they share occurs in the context of a real relationship. Some kind of relationship narrative, even if it is false, seems to make the sex act more satisfying. This wisdom has been taken up by futuristic sex-robot manufacturers. They understand the market importance of adding intimacy, companionship and conversation to sexual gratification in their sexbots and are investing a lot of money in making their tech more and more relatable (Sharkey et al., 2017.)

'If I just wanted to cum, I'd just masturbate at home. So it's nice to actually spend time with a girl (sex worker) and actually be able to make her feel nice as well. Like part of the enjoyment for me is feeling like I've actually made her day too, and I try my best to do that … When you do a full service sometimes you're just about to go and kiss her and she'll be like, "I'm sorry, I don't do kissing". In my head I've just forced myself upon her and it makes me embarrassed. It's very mechanical, and it feels a bit more like a transaction I guess because you really are just giving her money to please yourself.' – **Dave**

Despite the ready availability of "meaningless" sex, most people have an eventual goal of forming a committed relationship. Research has found that many people even use hook-ups to try to achieve this (Weitbrecht & Witton, 2017). They also find that the rise in hook-ups has not meant the demise of relationships in college populations. In one study, 74% of college women reported they had been in a relationship that lasted at least six months (Armstrong et al., 2012).

Dr Helen Fisher, relationship researcher and adviser for the dating website Match.com, suggests that rather than sex being devoid of meaning, the current trend is one of "slow love". She speculates that before marriage, people are taking time to sleep around, have friends with benefits, or live with their partners. However, she believes that no matter how culture shifts or choices change, romantic attachment and forming a pair bond is most people's ultimate aim (Fisher, 2016).

Indeed, a 2012 survey found that 83% of men and 84% of women said that having a successful marriage was still "one of the most important things" or "very important" in life (Pattern & Parker, 2012). As such, even though the pleasures of the flesh are more readily available and more culturally endorsed, the drive to connect, to bond, to feel love – or at least to feel something more than fleeting sexual pleasure – remains a primary human process that most aim to satisfy at some point.

'We hooked up in a club. Then I saw her at another club, and we hooked up again. Then, we started deliberately going to clubs, intending to hook up with one another.

'We didn't even speak of a relationship, or want to go for a date; we were at a stage where we wanted to just have fun, and we were

very attracted to each other. A few months of this, and we started talking to one another more regularly. A little under a year after our first hook-up she told me, "We can't keep on doing this – it either has to go somewhere, or we need to stop." I thought about it for all of five seconds – and it was only that long because I was drunk. We went on a date the following week. I have been with her for over nine years now and got married last autumn.' – **Trent**

FOR THE LOVE OF A VOLE

Strangely enough, most of what we know about romantic attachment, pair bonding and love in humans has come from a little rodent called the prairie vole. Unlike 97% of mammals, prairie voles are monogamous and form very strong attachments to one another. In cute coincidence, the word *vole* is, after all, an anagram for *love*.

A male vole will court the female so that she goes into oestrus (the rodent equivalent of ovulation). They mate in passionate forty-hour sessions. And, during this process and the hours that follow, they bond for life – male voles will stick around to raise babies. And when a vole's partner dies, voles experience something akin to grief.

The hormones responsible for attachment in these animals are oxytocin and vasopressin, both of which are released during sex. Studies show that when male voles are given a dose of vasopressin, or females of oxytocin, the animals bond on sight with the nearest potential mate, before sex even occurs. Interestingly, prairie-vole sex involves an unusual amount of vaginal-cervical stimulation – probably an adapted behaviour that triggers the oxytocin release.

In humans, oxytocin is released for women (and to a lesser extent men) from prolonged eye contact, nipple stimulation and orgasm. Vasopressin is associated with male arousal. As such, whether you are male or female, human sex encourages attachment and love and it could be argued that, just like the prairie vole, we are not designed to have sex without forming some sort of attachment.

EXERCISE: FINDING YOUR "WHY?"

What role does sex play in your life? If we had a crystal ball and told you that you will never have sex again, what would you lose?

Are some types of sex better than others for you? Is that because of what happens physically during the sex or something else?

Have you had "meaningless" sex before? Was it a good experience?

In some kink practices it is commonplace for each participant to share their intentions for the experience they are about to create before they begin. Next time you begin to be sexual (with a partner or by yourself) think about identifying and perhaps even sharing your intentions for the experience before beginning.

PART 2: SUMMARY AND EXERCISES

In current times, where sex for the sake of sex is permissible, graphic sex is everywhere in the media and watching porn is a common pastime, we absorb many sexpectations. Whether you relate to the sexpectations we have described above or not, what is more important is that your reading of them has made you more conscious about your beliefs about sex and "good sex", and whether they are helping or hindering you.

To recap, the sexpectations we have explored (which are by no means an exhaustive list!) are:

- It is "normal" to identify as either as a "man" or a "woman", to be heterosexual and to want a monogamous relationship that should develop along a standard trajectory known as the "Relationship Escalator".
- Picking a sexual partner, especially a committed, long-term sexual relationship, should be predicated on feeling some "chemistry" and physical attraction.
- Desire is an essential precursor to sex, and that sexual desire is ideally high, well matched and reliable in a long-term relationship – though we also paradoxically expect desire to fade in a long-term relationship.
- Men are biologically more "horny" than women and they are more happy to have meaningless or casual sex.

- Sex doesn't really count unless PIV is involved.
- The natural conclusion of the sexual act is orgasm and that both partners should experience orgasm at least once during a sexual event.
- We should all be sexually adventurous, sexually skilled, and have great bodies – like porn stars.
- It's okay and even desirable to have meaningless sex.

If you were to pick just one sexpectation (it could be one of these or a new one) that you think has the biggest negative influence on your sexual satisfaction, which would it be?

What would you have to believe in this area of your sex life to feel more satisfied? Rewrite the sexpectation as if it was written to suit you.

Think back to past partners and past difficult or disconnected sexual experiences – can you see the influence of any unhelpful sexpectations in them now?

Think about how you might be unconsciously perpetuating your sexpectations with your sexual partners and also in your social conversations. What would it mean to not take these beliefs for granted and instead to approach them with curiosity and as more of an option rather than a necessity?

PART 3

DISCOVERING WHAT YOU REALLY WANT

[Your Guide to Embodied Sexuality]

CHAPTER 14

A NEW TAKE ON SEXPERTISE

Nowadays there are many books, magazine articles and YouTube instructional videos which will endeavour to teach us how to have better sex, be a better lover, last longer, cum harder... Yet few of these are genuinely helpful. Sure, we may pick up a "tip" or two, and we may stumble across one author who seems to write from a place we can relate to. However, because of the myriad of sexpectations we all carry, most of this well-meaning advice will be riddled with assumptions that are likely to either not reflect our experience or be helpful for us. Assumptions based on heteronormativity, PIV or orgasm being essential components of sex, about our motivations for sex ... In fact, all the sexpectations we outlined in Part 2 and many more are represented both in the popular and academic sex advice available. In a way, this advice creates the problem it is trying to fix by reinforcing narrow ideas about what "good sex" is, and increasing our pressure to conform and perform.

As such, in this book we will not be going over different sex positions but instead be helping you tune in to how your body wants to be positioned, to be touched and to move. We will not be prescribing to you what makes for "better" sex, as if sex is a one-size-fits-all experience. Instead, we will help you with being present in your body to allow yourself to discover what works uniquely for you. And, of course, by raising awareness of the habitual sexpectations that have been stuck in your head, we will have given you a method for breaking free of them so you can have the sex you *really* want.

The process of getting what you *really* want can be simplified into three skill sets: getting unstuck from your head; becoming present in your body; and communicating well. These steps are simple enough to learn and, with practice, can become an effortless and automatic approach to sexual situations.

To begin this process you will need to become familiar with the sensation of sexual energy. "Sexual energy" is a term I borrow from the Tantric tradition, but you can think of sexual energy as arousal – the feeling in your body when you are "turned on". Sexual energy does not reference a particular stage of Kaplan's sexual response cycle (see Chapter 8) (such as the "arousal" phase) and is not therefore a specific "level" of sexual energy, but rather a more nuanced sensation that changes in feeling and intensity over the course of a sexual experience.

You might experience sexual energy as a heat that flushes through your body, you might feel it as a tingling or swelling in your genitals, you might be more aware of excitement in your chest or your heart beating and breath quickening. Sexual energy gives you the feeling that tells you "I find this sexy" and it can be very subtle.

For example, a touch on the shoulder can comfort and reassure but may not stimulate any kind of sexual energy or awareness. Whereas, the same touch from another person – perhaps a new date, a crush, or maybe even a random stranger – can infuse you with a subtle awareness. This sense of alertness and feeling alive from that touch may be the first stirring of the sexual energy we are hoping to get you more connected with.

Another concept to become familiar with is "embodiment". Learning how to pay attention to and stay connected with your in-the-moment "embodied experience" means being fully present in your body and paying attention to the information it makes available to you in the form of sensations, sights, smells, tastes, sounds, energy, etc. Then, to remain embodied, you will need to learn how to stay tuned in to that information as it shifts over time.

Practising embodiment helps us better learn our own sexual responses, what stimulates and what subdues our sexual energy (our turn-ons and turn-offs), and how to stay connected with ourselves both over the course of one discrete sexual experience, but also as our body changes over months and years. It is only when we can stay present in and track our experience that we can truly understand our preferences and our boundaries and help our partners give us the best sex we can have.

Also, when we learn how to stay present in our embodied experience and communicate our needs from that place, we are in the best place to show any interested partner how to better communicate with us about their own sexual needs. And, even if they don't develop the comfort to communicate verbally with us, the heightened bodily awareness we have cultivated within ourselves will assist us in becoming more sensitive to their bodily responses – which is another great source of information. Developing this communication and sensitivity will, in turn, increase your confidence and ability to stimulate their sexual energy and give them what works for them.

However, we want to acknowledge that not everybody does want more sexpertise or better sex and that that choice is fine. You can have sex if you want to, but you certainly don't have to have sex. People differ a lot in terms of their interest in sex and plenty of people and relationships are perfectly happy and healthy without any sex or with having perfunctory or "good-enough" sex.

Some of the people who might relate to this (but not all people in these categories do!) are sex workers who just want to do their job, people who are asexual or not interested in sex themselves and may, or may not, want to provide it to their partners, and people who have experienced sexual abuse. We want people to be whoever they are and do whatever they need to do without judgement. For everyone ready to explore, however, it can be transformational to make best friends with your body and listen to it for information, even and especially when things get awkward, anxiety-provoking or uncertain.

FROM SEXPECTATIONS TO SEXPERTISE

Our sexpectations often materialise in unhelpful thoughts about sex in daily life and also specifically during sex. Because of this, we can unnecessarily limit ourselves or overextend past our bodies' consent. Only you can be the expert on your experiences, your body and your desires. No culturally endorsed sexpectations will ever give you "better sex" unless you check in with your body to see if you are indeed enjoying what the sexpectation prescribes.

For example, there is nothing inherently bad about penetration or orgasm – it's just not what your body will feel like doing *all* the time or *every* time (and for some people at *any* time!). When we let go of these preconceived sexpectations, we can tune in to what actually works for us to create and build our own sexual energy.

Most of us have probably had an experience where one kind of erotic or sexual activity worked for us really well on one occasion, but not as well on another. For example, you might have had a similar blow job from the same partner that was great one time, but another time left you cold.

If you think about the differences between these experiences – the situations, the feelings, the sensations, the thoughts – you will understand why a one-size-fits-all approach will never work when it comes to sex. In sex, it isn't *what* you do, it's *how* you do it. So, when we are preoccupied with sexpectations, we focus on what we "should" do and feel. But when we are concentrating on what works for us, the emphasis is much more on how we really *want* to touch and be touched.

The differences you might identify between sexual activities that work and don't work for you are listed below. They will roughly fall into three overlapping categories: whether you get stuck in your head, whether you are present to your body, and whether you are communicating well for connection and consent. These map on to the three skill sets necessary for true "sexpertise" that we will detail in the following chapters. Because ultimately, great sex is about being present and embodied, and communicating what you want.

EXERCISE: SPOT THE DIFFERENCE

Thinking back to your example of a sexual experience that worked well one time and not well another, answer the following questions:

Stuck in your head?

- Were you comparing yourself to other people or an ideal in your head?
  'I was thinking I was not as good as their ex.'
- Were you focused on your partner's experience?
  'I was wondering if I was being too rough for her.'
- Were you being critical about yourself or others?
  'I was thinking that I must look terrible in this position.'
- Were you focused on your performance or what you "should" be doing?
  'I was telling myself that I shouldn't make those sounds!'
- How focused were you on achieving a goal as opposed to enjoying the journey?
  'I was wondering if I would cum this time?'

Present in your body?

- How "in the moment" or "present" were you?
  'I was thinking about what would happen next.'
- How aware of your sensations were you?
  'I could feel his breath on my neck.'
- How much sexual energy did you notice? Did it change over the experience?
  'As I was about to cum, I felt intense tingles in my fingers and toes.'

Communicating well?

- How consensual did it feel to you?
  'I felt like I was doing it for them, rather than for me.'
- How connected did you feel with anyone else involved?
  'It felt like we were having two completely separate experiences.'

- How confident were you that it was working for your partner?

  'I wasn't sure if she came.'
- How much feedback did you give and receive?

  'He made no sounds at all – I had no idea if he was having a good time.'
- How many requests did you make and receive? If someone said no, how did that go down?

  'She sulked for the rest of the night when I said I wasn't up for that.'

CHAPTER 15

STUCK IN YOUR HEAD

WHERE DID IT COME FROM?

We begin our journeys of becoming stuck in our heads early in life. As children we learn to override the signals of our body and follow social convention so we can "fit in", be liked, loved and accepted. We are taught to deny, ignore or suppress our body's impulses, boundaries and preferences. Don't cry, be quiet. Don't cling, be independent. Don't like the taste of vegetables? Eat them anyway, they are good for you. Don't like Aunty? Be polite and give her a hug anyway. Does touching your genitals feel good? Get your hand out of there! Pretty girl? Don't stare. Don't want to have sex anymore? But you said you would and he'll be disappointed if you don't …

These messages all add together to foster the belief that the body is not acceptable as it is and is not to be trusted or listened to. As such, we all learn to dissociate from our bodies and treat them with suspicion and contempt rather than the unconditional love, respect and acceptance they deserve. It is this love, this "friendship" that we need to cultivate with our bodies that is the basis of "self-esteem" – and we all know how much easier it is to navigate the relational and sexual world when we have good self-esteem!

As the old saying goes: "you can't love anyone else until you love yourself". Only when we apply the actions of love to our bodies – as if our bodies were indeed our "best friends" – are we are able to receive love from others. These loving actions – paying attention and listening; treating ourselves kindly; responding to our needs; and protecting our boundaries – will furnish us with the insight we need to show up with others and be truthful about who we are and what we need. Being authentic in this way allows them to pay loving attention and listen to our real selves, treat us kindly, be responsive and honour our boundaries. Take these examples:

> *Kaylene was tired and really didn't feel like having sex. But she had put Bill off last time and she didn't want to let him down again. Bill could sense something was off with Kaylene; she seemed a little flat and distracted. He had asked her if everything was okay and, she said she was fine, so he tried his hardest to please her and do the things he knew she liked. On the way home Kaylene fumed to herself, 'That self-absorbed idiot! All he wants from me is sex!' She resolved not to see him again.*

Compared with:

> *Kaylene was tired and really didn't feel like having sex. She felt guilty that she had put Bill off last time and saying no again might disappoint him. However, she knew she needed to listen to her body and get an early night. Her responsibility to meet her own needs far outweighed her responsibility to meet whatever she might imagine Bill's needs to be! She said to Bill, 'I'm really tired and I think I*

just need to go home.' Bill was surprised and disappointed but very happy to let her do what she needed to do; he cared about her and he certainly didn't want to have sex if she wasn't into it.

In the first example, Kaylene is stuck in her own head, stuck in the ideas of "right" and "wrong", "should" and "should not". She allows these thoughts to dictate what she does and, in doing so, ignores her body and steps out of consent with herself.

All of us do this to some extent. We eat beyond fullness, or don't eat enough, or don't eat what our body is truly craving. We ignore our tired eyes and yawns, only sleeping when our work is done or our TV show is over. We push through pain to achieve our goals and don't notice physical discomfort until it is so significant we need to take painkillers. We struggle to be present and may rely on fantasy during sex, or get lost in other thoughts, and then complain about how empty and mediocre our sex life seems, becoming obsessed with what we should be feeling but surprised when we feel unfulfilled.

THE HEAD GAME

Sex is often a "head game" when it should be the domain of the body – we could say we are often "fucked" in the head! In our modern world, with all its desk jobs and smartphones, we are very good at being in our head. Being in our head can be useful in daily life – we'd never solve problems or answer emails if we didn't spend *some* time up there! However, it is rarely useful during sex. The types of thoughts that get us caught up in our heads during sex can loosely be divided into: distraction, time travelling, spectatoring and self-criticism.

The key to getting unfucked in the head is to become aware of which of these habitual unhelpful thinking habits pop up regularly for you. These particular thoughts often come up again and again, so, because they are so familiar, it can be relatively easy to identify them. Rather than focus on them or follow what they would have you do in the moment, thank your mind for them and let them go. Then, bring your attention back to the sensations of your body and what it is telling you.

'I know the thought I most struggle with, my "inner critic", is very vocal! Every time I have sex it tells me that I have a small cock and I'll never satisfy my partner. It used to make me avoid penetration and sometimes I focused so much on how small I was I'd lose my erection and get even smaller! Nowadays, the thoughts still come up for me but I'm getting good at brushing them away and refocusing my attention on what I'm doing with my partner and how good it feels.' – **Mark**

Distraction is one of the most recognisable ways of getting stuck in our heads during sex. Some of us get distracted because we have a lot of stress, so we find our mind wandering off to solve problems or to worry whenever it is not thinking about other things. Others find that staying focused on one thing and clearing their mind is more difficult in general, independent of what is happening for them in life. In a terrible irony, some men even use distraction (e.g. remembering shopping lists!) to help reduce their levels of sexual energy so that they can last longer during sex – *do not* try this at home! The old saying "lie back and think of England" is another (horrible!) example of using distraction to endure sex. There are plenty of more skilful ways of managing your sexual energy.

Time travelling is when we go forwards or back in time in our minds. When we go forwards in time, we are usually focused on a goal. For example, a man who is performing oral sex might be time travelling to the PIV he is hoping to get to next, and not on the oral experience. Similarly, some people think about when the sex will be over whilst they are still having it! We can also time travel backwards and ruminate on things that have occurred earlier. We often think about the bad or embarrassing things that have happened in this way. For example, if we clash teeth when kissing or a man loses his erection, these memories can keep bubbling up and catching our attention even when the sexual experience has moved on.

Spectatoring, as mentioned before, involves focusing from a third-person perspective on how we look, how we sound or how we are performing rather than focusing on our bodily experience. Magazines, movies and social media bombard us with idealised and airbrushed images and what we see in the mirror (particularly in *certain* positions!) rarely lives up to them. Additionally, focusing on how we think we look and the judgements that we imagine our partners make of us (which are more accurately a projection of our own self-criticism) leads to self-consciousness, shame and anxiety – not very sexy emotions!

We also tend to be the umpires of our own performance when spectatoring. We constantly compare our performance to past experiences, porn, our own ideals and sexpectations or our imaginings of what our partner wants. This preoccupation with how we think we are measuring up actually makes us *worse* in bed because it limits our ability to pay attention to the experience we are having and the cues our partner is giving us in the present. Paying attention to our own performance is also unlikely to build our sexual energy and turn us on – it can therefore create the performance problems we are so desperate to avoid! As I say to my clients with erection difficulties, thinking about your own penis during sex is not really going to do it for you!

Spectatoring occurs because we want to excel; we want to look good and be good in bed because we believe that this will gain us admiration, respect, love and protect us from rejection. Some of us are so concerned with how our partners view us that we become completely focused on trying to please them and lose touch with ourselves, our own needs and feelings and step way beyond our boundaries.

Self-criticism is a close bedfellow (excuse the pun!) of spectatoring. When we are focused on our looks and our performance, we are bound to find something that we don't like. It is easy then to get caught up in internally berating ourselves (once again, *not* a sexy experience for most of us!). We call ourselves names, go over and over our perceived flaws or what we "should" have done differently, imagine the critical thoughts of our partners and imagine the terrible future consequences that might occur. The ways we can be our own worst critic are many and varied.

COMMON UNHELPFUL THINKING PATTERNS IN SEX

Should-ing and Must-ing

Applying inflexible rules and standards to your actions.

> *I should go down on him because he went down on me.*
>
> *I shouldn't ask him to cuddle me afterwards, it's only a hook-up.*

Black-and-white Thinking

Thinking in terms of all or nothing.

> *It's not really sex unless we have PIV.*
>
> *Unless I make her cum I've failed.*

Overgeneralisation

Thinking that because something happened in the past (or hasn't happened) it will or should always happen (or not happen).

'I never cum from oral so don't even bother.'

'She always says no whenever I come on to her.'

Negative Mental Filtering

Focusing on the negative details at the expense of any positive.

'My cellulite will be terrible in this position.'

"He wasn't very loud when he came, maybe he didn't have a good time."

Labelling and Criticising

Attacking ourselves with critical names and negative judgements.

'My vulva is ugly and deformed!'

'I'm a bad lay, I can't perform like the porn stars I watch.'

Catastrophisation

Making mountains out of molehills (making a bigger deal out of something than it calls for).

'If I have sex with another guy, I'll turn gay.'

'What if the condom had a rip in it? I could have HIV!'

Mind Reading

Assuming you know what someone else is thinking.

'She'll think I'm perverted if I ask for that.'

'She's tired, she won't want sex now.'

Fortune Telling

Assuming you can predict the future.

'If I don't do anal, he'll ghost me.'

'When we get married, we won't have sex anymore.'

Personalisation

Blaming yourself for everything that goes wrong.

'She wasn't very wet, maybe I didn't give her enough foreplay.'

'He wanted sex last time but said no this time — have I pissed him off?'

CHAPTER 16

BEING PRESENT AND EMBODIED

EXERCISE: PAYING ATTENTION TO YOUR NEW BODY BFF
Before we get this chapter started, I invite you to take a deep breath, and notice how it feels to inhabit your body in this moment. Is there an immediate unmet need? Could you take care of it before reading on further?

For example:

- Do you need water or other hydration?
- Are you at the right temperature or do you need a blanket or a fan?
- Are you as comfortable as you could be in the position you are sitting?
- How hungry are you? Do you need food, if so what is your body craving?
- How fatigued are you? Do you need a break or a nap?

Paying attention to your body in the way you have just done is key to developing your sexpertise. When you were paying attention, you focused on the present moment – you had what we call "presence". With presence during sex you will be able to notice more details, be more responsive and more flexible to suit your (and any partner's) needs.

In the above exercise you also experienced "embodiment". As discussed before, embodiment is a form of presence where your awareness is rooted in your physical experience – the sensations, sights, smells, tastes, sounds, etc. This is in contrast to, for example, mindfulness of your thoughts, where you are present but your attention is on what comes to mind, rather than what your body is experiencing. It sounds tricky, but never fear – these two elements of presence in the moment and awareness of your body can be trained!

Because of the sexpectations that get stuck in our heads, sex is often the most challenging experience to be present to. As we explored in the previous chapter, we often have our inner critic hating on our bodies, a lot of "shoulds" about what we should do and what we shouldn't do floating around our minds, and we become focused on the goal (e.g. getting her off, staying hard) rather than enjoying the journey. As such, it's often useful to first train these skills outside of a sexual situation and build up to practising them whilst you are having sex. We will give you some exercises to help you do this below.

As a general rule, the easiest place to start with practising presence and embodiment is during physical activities that don't involve anyone else. For example, as you gradually dissolve a piece of chocolate on your tongue or whilst you are brushing your teeth. Then, when you are ready, you can try your skills during solo masturbation or sexual self-touch. Once you feel you can be present and embodied there you are ready to graduate to involving the touch of others in a non-sexual way. For example, you could try your skills of being present and embodied when receiving a non-sexual massage. The next step might be trying these skills during a sensual kiss but try not to jump ahead to the thought of "what might happen next?" but stay with the kiss and savour it for its own sake … and, of course, eventually we want you to try out these skills during partnered sex, as well!

As you practise, you will notice thoughts and external distractions bubble up. You will also notice your mind running ahead (to what will happen next or a specific goal) or back (to what just happened or happened before) – both points of focus that will pull you out of presence. This will happen *every* time, to *every* person – you are not doing it incorrectly!

When you notice these thoughts (e.g. *Does my bum look big?*) and external distractions (e.g. voices in another room), try to practise what is known as "nonattachment". Allow yourself to notice what you notice without judgement, or labelling it or yourself as good or bad. Then, let it go and refocus your attention on your body and other aspects of your sexual experience (e.g. the feeling of connection, the hardness of her nipples, the pulse in his cock).

In this approach we put the information made available to you through your body – the awareness of feelings or sensations, sights, sounds, tastes, sexual energy – in a different category to the thoughts and distractions described above. These are the sensations we want you to focus on as they unfold, and this is the awareness that we want you to bring your attention back to when it wanders. This is embodiment. We use this awareness of the feelings and sensations to anchor our attention in the present moment. They will also guide us on how we would like to progress the sexual experience and build our sexual energy (if we would like to!).

As modern life becomes increasingly disembodied, with all its screens and demands on our attention, it can be hard to even know where to begin when trying to open up your awareness of yourself. To help you out, below is some guidance through three simple exercises of embodied focus that you can use to become more body aware, more present in the moment, and more open to sensory experience.

EXAMPLE EMBODIMENT EXERCISES

1. NOTICE YOUR BREATH

Arrange yourself in a comfortable position. Close your eyes and allow the sounds of the room to wash over you as you begin to focus inwards. Notice your next gentle inhale. You might like to focus on the sensation of the air running over your top lip or between your lips, or you could focus on the sensation of your nostrils filling. Alternatively you might prefer to notice the sensation of your lungs filling from the inside, or your chest rising from the outside. There is no right or wrong, and you are welcome to dance your attention across all these different points of focus and others at any time during this experience. Perhaps you find one point of focus more soothing or works better for you than others?

You can notice the rhythm of your breathing. Notice the pause between your inhale and your exhale. Just notice that moment in between. As you inhale now, see if you can just notice the inhalation, like a curious observer, and not try to change it or control it. Now, see if you can do the same for your exhalation. You can notice your breath for as long or as short a time as you wish.

Even a moment of body awareness is a moment spent in the present, not lost in concerns about the past or plans for the future. Every time you notice your attention wander to the past or future, other thoughts or distractions, just notice, without judgement, and gently bring your attention back to the breath sensations.

2. FIND YOUR PELVIC FLOOR

In Tantric traditions they used breath and pelvic-floor contraction and release to build sexual energy and move it around the body. They even believed that sexual energy could jump from one body to the other! Good muscular strength in your pelvic floor is important for good sexual performance because it is those muscles that pump the blood into your genitals. Blood in your genitals makes them more sensitive, more turgid (erect) and brings more oxygenated "buzz" to them (just think of the "pins and needles" you get when blood rushes back to your legs after you have been sitting on them – kind of orgasmic, eh?). This is the less sexy, modern medicalised explanation for the Tantrika's experience of "sexual energy".

Although the contraction exercises we are about to do *are* important for strength and good sexual performance, that is not our aim in giving you them. Instead, we want you to use them as a way to begin to pay more exquisite attention to the area of your pelvic bowl and your genitals. In our culture this is a taboo and hidden area of the body. We have to cover it with clothes at all times, we aren't allowed to touch it, smell it and heaven forbid we feel it at inappropriate times!

So, go ahead and arrange yourself in a comfortable position. Close your eyes and allow the sounds of the room to wash over you as you begin to focus inwards. Drift your attention down to your pelvis and genitals. Become aware of any sensations available to you. Perhaps you can feel the cloth of your underwear. Perhaps you can feel warmth. Perhaps you can notice the sensations in different parts of your genitals – your penis, your testes, your clitoris, your vagina, your anus. Perhaps you notice a gentle "vitality" or energy …

Become aware of your pubococcygeus (PC) muscle, also known as "Kegels". These are the muscles near your genitals that also control the flow of urine through your urethra. So, imagine you need to stop the flow of urine mid-flow – your PC muscles are the ones you would squeeze to do this.

With your next inhale gently squeeze these muscles up. Then, in your natural breath rhythm, with your next exhale gently release these muscles. Notice the feelings in your pelvis and genitals as you go through around ten rounds of breath (or to the point of fatigue). Perhaps you can feel more warmth, more energy, perhaps not. Perhaps you can notice the muscles get tired and less responsive – that's okay! It's normal and will improve with practice.

When you have finished, just relax and observe the sensations in your pelvic bowl. If you are not too tired, begin another round of breath and squeezing and then pause again and observe. Do as many rounds as is comfortable, remembering that if this practice is new to you, you will need to go gently and ease into it with short sessions – your PC muscles get sore from a workout like this, just like any other muscles in your body!

3. BODY SCAN

Arrange yourself in a comfortable position sitting or lying down. It's a good idea to close your eyes to help you focus.

When you do so, you may notice the sounds in the room and you can allow them to wash over you. You can then draw your attention inwards to your body.

You might like to start by noticing the top of your head. How does the top of your head feel? Does your scalp feel tight or relaxed? Does your scalp have a temperature? Can you feel the hair on your scalp? Whatever the answer, don't try to change it – just notice it. Imagine you're scanning your way down your body slowly. Notice the back of the head. Now towards the ears, then to the face. Can you feel any sensations on the skin of your face? You might like to feel for the smoothness of your forehead. You might like to feel the weight of your eyelids as they rest closed. Work your way down. Notice your jaw, is it loose or does it carry tension?

If your attention wanders to thoughts of why, for example, your jaw is the way it is, and you're suddenly off in a story about something that happened to you, or some judgement of it being the way it is, acknowledge this but don't berate yourself for it. Just gently return to noticing your body.

Notice your neck and how your head sits on top of it. Notice your shoulders, and so on. In this way, slowly scan down your body all the way to your feet, to the very ends of your toes. You might like to imagine the body as having an "internal landscape" of sensation. Different parts feeling differently. You can notice the surface sensations on your skin and the deep sensations of your muscles, organs and bones. You may notice some emotions in certain parts of your body.

Some parts of your body may be more enjoyable to notice for you than other parts and that is totally okay. If you'd like to, you can just stick with your favourite parts, or you might like to challenge yourself and gently lean into sensations that work less well for you, knowing you can stop at any time, respecting your own limits.

If you can give ten or fifteen minutes to this practice, great! If you can't, even a couple of minutes of body scanning can help to bring more awareness to the body, slow the heart rate, and bring a greater sense of calmness and clarity.

CHAPTER 17

SEXUAL SELF-TOUCH DONE RIGHT

We've all heard the warnings: masturbation will make you blind, your penis might fall off … you might even be sentenced to hell! To this day, many adults have early experiences of being shamed for touching their genitals as a child. Because of the shame around masturbation and fear of being "caught" in the act, many men learn early on to masturbate quickly and efficiently with the sole goal of orgasm. For the same reasons, and perhaps also because of the anatomy of female genitals being more "inside" and therefore less obvious and easy to explore, many women never learn to masturbate.

In our PIV-obsessed world, where sex is considered not to "count" unless it involves PIV, masturbation can be seen as "pathetic", an act for lonely losers who can't get partnered sex. In hetero relationships, it can be positioned as anything from unnecessary (because if you have access to PIV, you'd want that, surely?) to a betrayal of trust.

However, masturbation can be a very useful and important practice. How can we explain to another person what works effectively for our bodies, if we don't know ourselves? As a result, often the touch that we receive from other people is not what really works for us. Masturbation provides the best opportunity to explore the sensations of different touch with curiosity, and to notice how our sexual energy responds.

Because of the sexpectations around orgasm – that it is the proper destination of any sexual act – many people think that orgasm is the sole goal of masturbation. They also therefore think that masturbation only involves the touching of the genitals. We have nothing against orgasm nor genitals. Yet, once again, when you are overly focused on the goal of orgasm, you can lose the enjoyment of the full bodily experience of touch and sexual energy. Similarly, when you are only focused on the genitals, you don't learn the many things that might work for you when other parts of your body are touched.

In order for us to bypass the mental default that "masturbation" refers to genital touch only, from here on we will refer to it as "sexual self-touch." Sexual self-touch enables us to notice what our bodies like so that we can better ask for what we want. It also improves the skilfulness of the touch that we ourselves give. In giving ourselves time, presence and responding to what our body needs with our touch, we grow in our capacity to give this type of touch to others.

BREAKING UNHELPFUL HABITS

To distinguish sexual self-touch from genitally focused, goal-directed, quick and functional masturbation we recommend:

1. **Setting an intention** – it could be "to go slowly", "stay present", "stay in my body and not get lost in the porn".

2. **Take your time** – set aside ten to thirty minutes to immerse yourself in your experience.

3. **Become aware of and experiment with breath, sound and movement** – Self-touch for orgasm usually involves holding the breath, no sound and minimal body movement. Breathing consciously, making sound and encouraging movement contribute to the feedback loop that builds sexual energy.

4. **Savour** – it's okay if you orgasm (as long as you weren't rushing it!) and it's also okay if you don't. Either way, after your experience take a few minutes to breathe and to notice the sensations in your body. Give yourself the space to savour the experience so you can integrate it in your body and embed it in your mind, which will help you change unhelpful habits.

There is a huge variety in the types of sexual self-touch that work for different people. For example, some people need wetness, others dry friction. Some use hands, others rub against a pillow, or use the water flowing out of a shower head. Some people like to use vibrators during sexual self-touch, and in this too there is huge variation around what people like. In terms of sensation, some like suction, others gentle stroking, others need a really firm pressure … You get the picture: there are as many variations in sexual self-touch as there are people who touch themselves!

It is common for people to find that they have one very effective way of touching themselves. When we find something that works for us, it's easy to just do that thing over and over. Although it's important to listen to our bodies and what builds sexual energy for us, it is also useful and interesting to try other things as well. So, for example, if you always use sex toys, mixing it up with non-toy sexual self-touch is important as well. Try keeping an open mind and engaging in a variety of sensations, touches, pressures, positions etc. Going outside our regular habit can help us to explore what turns us on, and how our body works. Additionally, when we do the same thing again and again, there can be a number of negative things that can happen:

1. It can become more "automatic" and we can tend towards losing presence and embodiment as a result.
2. We can develop unhelpful thoughts about what works for us and what doesn't, which might be an overly narrow range or become outdated over time.
3. We can train our bodies to respond more efficiently to certain sensations and not others, thereby limiting the enjoyment we could have in other acts and sensations.

For example, there are people with a penis who always grip themselves so firmly and without lube during masturbation that they find it hard to stay erect or come to orgasm during PIV. Their partner's vagina provides very different sensations and pressure to what they are used to. Similarly, if people with vaginas get overly used to bringing themselves to orgasm with a particular vibration, they often struggle to orgasm when they are with a male partner. Penises feel very different from vibrators!

Joseph Kramer, the creator of the practice of sexological bodywork (a therapeutic touch based modality used to heal sexual issues), recommends that we touch ourselves in different positions (sitting, standing, lying down, etc.) to combat the potentially negative effect of conditioning our body to only respond sexually in our "porn position" (i.e. the body position we watch porn in). Dr Kramer also recommends a practice he calls the "porn pendulum" for sexual self-touch whilst watching porn. In this practice we alternate between watching porn to build our arousal/ sexual energy and looking away or pausing it to focus on our bodily sensations and our self-touch. In doing so we begin to introduce more awareness of body sensation and counteract the negative effect porn can have of disconnecting us from our embodied experience.

EXERCISE: SELF-ASSESSMENT ON YOUR SEXUAL SELF-TOUCH

Think back to the last time you experienced sexual self-touch. What do you remember about the experience? Was it slow and pleasurable, or quick and functional? Was it different from the time before that in any way, or do you usually do it in the same way?

If someone else was sexual with you in the way you are sexual with yourself, do you think you would consider them a good lover? What do you think would happen to your sexual excitement and interest if you always had partnered sex the same way every time?

THE ROLE OF FANTASY

Content warning: Sexual-assault fantasy is mentioned without detail below.

Fantasy can be an important part of many people's sexual experiences and for those that it works for, it is a creative, fun and safe way to explore taboos. However, it can also become a way of disconnecting from our bodies and our sexual partners, and a way of getting stuck into unhelpful, habitual ways of turning on.

In the wake of *Fifty Shades of Grey* and the increased interest in kink, many people think that fantasies have to be really racy and wild. But, like everything else sexual, the fantasies that turn people on can be many and varied. Fantasies are simply the things that stimulate sexual energy when you think about them. A fantasy can be mundane or very psychologically meaningful. Just as psychotherapists sometimes invite people to reflect on their dreams, fantasies can sometimes tell us a lot about our hopes and fears and can also be a way of dealing with past trauma.

POPULAR CATEGORIES OF SEXUAL FANTASIES:

- **Role playing**
  We pretend to be certain characters such as a doctor and nurse, student and teacher, sex worker and client, owner and pet.
- **Specific sexual behaviours**
  This includes things like threesomes, oral sex, being spanked, being bound, sex outdoors. Most of the kinky acts would fall into this category.

- **Power dynamics**
  We might be into the idea of letting one person be completely in control, and the other person completely submissive.
- **Partners**
  We might fantasise about having sex with a celebrity or a crush. We might fantasise about having sex with someone of a different gender to the gender we are usually attracted to.
- **Stories**
  We may have fantasies about finding a stranger in our bed, or having sex with Santa. Rape fantasies are also really common (and OK!)
- **Feelings**
  Many of us fantasise about certain feeling states: being confident and uninhibited, being scared and vulnerable, being swept off our feet and ravished.

It's important to remember that fantasies are just fantasies: they are in your mind, not reality. Many people fantasise about things they have no intention of ever acting out, nor would they even be tempted to act out if given the opportunity. Sexual fantasies are the same as non-sexual fantasies in this way – no matter how many times, or in how much vivid detail we imagine strangling our siblings, we'd never *actually* do it. Similarly, there is no need to be frightened or ashamed of any fantasy you might have that works for you. An analysis of twenty studies indicated that between 31% and 57% of women have rape fantasies

(Critelli & Bivona, 2008), so it's pretty common to fantasise about things you wouldn't actually want to happen!

> *'I felt ashamed because I knew on an intellectual level that rape is bad and should not be tolerated. Being spanked and called a "dirty girl" or having a guy cum over me should be degrading and a turn-off … I couldn't understand how I could find it erotic! I felt embarrassed and would never have talked about my fantasy life with my partner – I'm supposed to be a feminist! It wasn't until I realised that at the heart of it, I wanted to be wanted. I wanted to be desired so badly that my partner couldn't control himself and just had to take me. When I think about it, there was never any real feeling of fear or shame in my fantasies, just a feeling of being ravished …'* – **Libby**

> *'Lots of the scenarios play out in public places, back hallways, libraries, up against a wall – which is funny, because my real sex life (monogamous and fairly vanilla) is pretty much confined to my bedroom and occasionally the living-room couch. Usually I'm fantasising about sex with a stranger, or two strangers, usually a man, sometimes a hetero couple. I'm always imagining that there's something illicit about the situation. To that last point, I've harboured an intense intellectual and physical/emotional crush on an older married colleague for years now, and often return to that in my fantasies.'* – **Brianna**

It might be helpful to recognise that fantasies are just the adult version of play. Like little kids acting out being school teachers and pupils, or doctors and patients in their play, sexual fantasies allow an outlet for creativity and fun. Fantasies allow us to explore other aspects of ourselves and try on completely different roles, with no cost or commitment. They don't need to "mean" anything or say anything about us. No matter how weird we may think our fantasies make us – all you need to do is google your most shameful perversion and the internet will show you dozens of people who are exactly the same kind of weird!

So, if fantasy works for you, please fantasise freely and prolifically! Although it is almost the definition of getting lost in your head, this is the one space we would encourage it. Sure, the element of in-the-moment presence does not always apply here, but embodiment can. In the same way we described checking in with your body intermittently whilst watching porn (the "porn pendulum"), you can thoroughly enjoy a fantasy whilst also being super aware of your physical arousal and the sexual energy stimulated by it.

When having partnered sex involving fantasy, we heartily endorse talking out or acting out your fantasy in a consensual way with a partner. It can be a highly erotic and embodied experience, if you pay attention to your body and the experience at hand! However, using fantasy to help you get off during a sexual experience that is not working for you whilst your partner is none-the-wiser is never recommended. Getting lost in a favourite fantasy of fucking some superstar whilst having sex with your partner is just plain rude!

EXERCISE: FIND YOUR FANTASIES

If you need a little help to uncover your fantasies, here are some sources of inspiration.

Think back to the exercise in Chapter 5 where we asked you to think about your hottest memories of sex and your sexual values - does anything really stand out?

What are the hottest sex scenes you've read in books, seen in movies, on TV or in porn? What did you like about them?

If you had to write your own erotica, what themes would you include?

Below are some common sexual fantasies. Try ranking them in order of most appealing to least and then think about what it is about them that made you choose that order:

- being raped or being ravished
- role playing teacher and student
- sex with a stranger
- having a threesome
- watching someone else have sex
- being watched having sex
- anal sex
- submission – being tied up, teased and spanked
- domination – having total control over your partner

CHAPTER 18

PARTNERED SEX YOU REALLY WANT

BEING PRESENT WITH A PARTNER

Through solo sexual self-touch we can develop the skill to stay present with and track the sensations and sexual energy in our bodies. We can also explore what works and what doesn't in order to develop a greater understanding of our preferences and boundaries. This skill can be carried over to partnered sex. However, with partnered sex there is, naturally, at least one other body to pay attention to and so we should practise splitting our attention; part of us attending to our embodied experience and the other part being present to our partner's sounds, scents, bodily reactions and verbal communication. This can happen simultaneously or you may like to alternate between the two. Below are a few tips for doing this skilfully.

1. Beginner's Mindset

As mentioned before, to be present in our sexual interactions we need to get out of our heads and let go of the need to "perform" and, instead, become a curious and eager observer or explorer, as if it was a completely new experience. Embracing this "beginner's mindset" is as important in partnered sex as it is in solo sexual self-touch. Just as our own body has different needs and responses at different times, so too will our partners. No matter if we have been with our partner more than a hundred times, we can still be surprised and learn something new about what works for them if we stay curious.

If we can bring presence and attention to our partners' bodies without preconception, we are more able to pick up on subtle cues that help us understand what works for them. For example, someone who braces themselves against the wall during sex may appreciate the offer of their arms being held down; someone who makes a sharp inhale when you run your fingers lightly across their thigh is probably really sensitive there.

2. Finding Your Flow

By intensely focusing on the person you are touching, where you are touching and how, you can achieve a state of "flow" with a partner. A "flow" state is an experience where a person performing an activity is fully immersed in a feeling of energised focus, full involvement and enjoyment. In essence, flow is characterised by complete absorption in what we are doing, a merging of action and awareness, and a loss of reflective self-consciousness. It can even result in a loss of sense of space and time (Nakamura & Csikszentmihályi, 2001). People in flow will report awareness of things such as the warmth of their partner's skin, noticing their partner incline towards them, and types of extra-sensory feelings such as feeling as if their partner's body is willing them to do certain things in certain ways.

'Personally, being a top is a very different type of euphoria. Whilst being a submissive is euphoric, being a top results in connection, concentration, and heightened senses. Whilst my bottom is enjoying their feral state, I am considerably zoned in on their needs and desires but acting without the need of forethought in my actions. I get to the point where the sense of separation from my partner, us being separate beings, seems to blur.' – **Zac**

Similar to solo sexual self-touch, when we become aware of being somewhere other than the present, we can simply notice that, let it be, take a breath that's a little deeper and slower than usual, and bring our awareness back to our bodies and to the present moment. Depending on the circumstances, we might also be able to verbalise it with our partners – say that we "checked out" or lost connection for a moment there – but we're back now.

3. Resolve or Respect When you Have Baggage

Unresolved conflict, dislike and anxiety about the relationship amongst other emotions can result in our body shutting down sexually. Similarly, many other factors such as pain, fatigue, sickness and stress can also mean our body just isn't feeling it when a partner might initiate sex. Ensure that any issues that are relevant "in the now" are addressed. If they aren't, they will prove a barrier to connected touch and the only thing we can do to stay in consent with ourselves is to respect our body's "no" and communicate it kindly.

'We had a big disagreement because I wanted what was right for us and something that I knew I could afford with just my income and she wanted the house she liked because she loved it. Neither one of us were budging on which house we wanted. We ended up

getting into our first fight and I said that I'm buying the house that I like because it's right for the both of us. It's been five months since we moved in and we haven't had sex since. I've asked her many times, and she keeps saying she doesn't feel like it, she doesn't feel close to me anymore.' – **Sam**

4. Experiment with Eye Contact

Eye contact is a brilliant way to increase our presence in a moment and stay connected with our partners. Maintaining eye contact creates a calming, connected state of being and is thought to trigger oxytocin – the feel-good, love and bonding chemical. Even in strangers, research has found that staring into each other's eyes for two uninterrupted minutes resulted in increased feelings of passionate love for each other (Kellerman et al., 1989.) Eye contact has the additional neat side effect of helping us pick up on what's working for our partner. Although it's nice to close our eyes during partnered sex so we can focus on the sensations we're experiencing, it is also good to experiment with eye contact for these reasons.

'Eye gazing became a very important ingredient to my love life, allowing me to connect fully with my partner during sex and surrender into the power of "now", by opening the gates that would interlock my soul with his. I understand why keeping eye contact during sex can feel weird, funny, awkward, uncomfortable, wrong, revealing, intimidating. But I've come to find that it's an ingredient I need in my life.' – **Tabitha**

5. Go Slow

When a partner makes us an offer, taking a moment to notice what our bodies answer can help break any bad habits we've formed about giving more automatic, people-pleasing "yes"es. This type of automatic yes is very common. Many of us feel as if we should know our answer and what we want immediately, or that taking time to notice our real answer is somehow gauche, rude or suggests we aren't having a good time – so we say yes on autopilot. Slowing down is key to letting this automatic yes drop away. And, once it has faded, the real answer will become clear. It may still be a yes, but it will be a real embodied yes rather than an automatic one.

Slowing down the breath also activates the parasympathetic nervous system, which is responsible for the rest-and-relax response. Sharing slow, deep breaths in time with a partner can be a helpful way of connecting because it helps us calm down, which will assist us in getting out of our head. It also requires that we pay attention to our partner's body with presence in order to track and emulate their breath.

'For me, slow sex creates the deepest connection with my partner, and I feel nurtured, deeply loved. It feels like a timeless connection that allows us to explore with a sense of wonder and with new eyes every time, to the extent that I find it really easy to talk about it and I am very comfortable to ask what I want from my partner.'
– **May**

6. Accept Change
Another aspect of being present with a partner is noticing that things change. Many people get stuck in their "shoulds" and think that if they have said yes to something, they should go through with what they've agreed to. But this does not apply to sex. We can say yes (or no) and then change our mind even if we've already begun. In fact, it's utterly important that we communicate what's happening, so that we remain aligned and in consent with our body.

If we slip in to what becomes merely tolerating touch, we lose connection with ourselves and with our partner/s. Getting stuck in thinking about the other person, or not wanting to "make a fuss" can be habitual and will generally lead to our bodies closing down and us beginning to feel dissociated from our experience. We owe it to ourselves and our partners to notice our "yes"es and "no"s and track any changes in them so we can give authentic answers to requests and offers. Our partners also owe it to us and to themselves to respect and value those authentic answers.

'We were in a beautiful hotel room on the first day of our holiday. But, after a while, my boyfriend was having trouble getting off. We changed position, his thrusts became rougher, and it started to hurt. My boyfriend asked if I was okay and I couldn't truthfully say yes although I knew it would disappoint him. I think it was the strength of our relationship that helped me say, "No, not really." I knew that no matter how sexually frustrated he would be, it would be unkind to both of us to let him keep going. It would ruin our holiday and we were just at the beginning.'– **Amy**

BEING CLEAR ABOUT WHO THE TOUCH IS FOR

Most of us like seeing our partner be turned on and getting off. It gives us pleasure to give pleasure and this can create a positive feedback loop where each partner reciprocally gets off on the other's pleasure. However, basing our pleasure on our partner's experience of pleasure can also lead us to get stuck in our heads. A partner may begin to think, *I need to fake it so he/she is happy,* and we may lose our own enjoyment because we are so externally focused on our partner having a good time.

In heterosexual relationships, one of the most common dynamics that leads to disconnection is the following:

Cameron loved his partner and wanted her to have the best time possible in the bedroom. He spent a lot of time on foreplay, kissing, touching and going down on her, trying to please her. Sometimes he became a bit annoyed though, because despite all he did to make it good for her, she never seemed to be that grateful …

Kim also loved Cameron. She knew that sex was important and enjoyed being close to him in this way, but she wasn't always as horny as he was and didn't need to have an orgasm to have a good time. But she knew he liked taking his time and that he found her body sexy so she was happy to let him do what he wanted to please him. However, every so often she got a little bit exasperated that he seemed to turn every session into a sex marathon.

During any sexual experience, it is important to understand who the touch is for. Some partners resolve these issues by making agreements about who will be the focus of the touch on different occasions – 'This time we'll focus on what works for you and next time we'll focus on me.' Alternatively, with good communication, it is possible to redirect the intention of who the touch is for partway through any sexual experience – 'After you cum, I'd love it if you went down on me …'

When we think about who touch is for, we usually default to assuming that the person doing the touch (usually the more active participant) is the giver and the person being touched is the receiver. For example, if I do a blow job (BJ), I'm the giver and he is the receiver. If he brushes my hair, he's now the giver and I am the receiver. However, there are many situations where this misses the true dynamic. Take, for example, if I am performing a BJ because I *love* it – I'm using his body for my pleasure (and he's willingly allowing it because he wants to give me pleasure). In this dynamic, although I'm the active participant (the 'doer'), I'm also the one receiving the gift!

However, someone rubbing up against a stranger on a train is very different. They are doing the touching but it is not a gift! They are taking something for their own sexual gratification without permission or consent. Likewise, a foot rub done in the hope it might lead to sex is touch with an agenda; although the recipient is given the touch, could we honestly say it is completely "for them"?

Dr Betty Martin talks about this as the "direction of the gift". Learning to differentiate between "giving" touch to another person (also known as "serving") and "taking" touch for yourself, can lead to sex that works better for all partners. Her model – "The Wheel of Consent" – is most easily understood by looking at the diagram below.

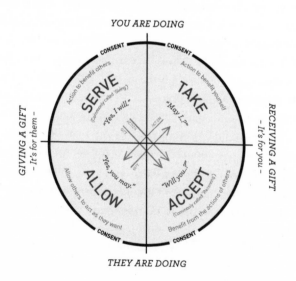

So, using my example above, if I am performing a BJ because I *love* it (i.e. it is for me), I am in the "taking" quadrant (top right) whereas, if I am doing it for his pleasure or because he requested one, I would be in the "serving" (or "giving") quadrant (top left). If a guy is letting me use his penis for a BJ (for *my* pleasure), he is in the "allowing" quadrant (bottom left), and if he is receiving the BJ (for *his* pleasure) he is in the bottom right quadrant – "accepting" (also known as "receiving").

EXERCISE: DANCING AROUND THE WHEEL

Looking at the different quadrants in the wheel on the previous page, have a go with your partner playing in the different roles.

When you are in the server/giver role ask: 'How would you like me to touch you?'

When you are in the accepter/receiver role say: 'Will you touch me [insert description]?'

When you are in the allower role say: 'How would you like to touch me?'

When you are in the taker role say: 'May I touch you like [insert description)]?'

Try to do this in an embodied way, when the touch is for you (i.e. you are the receiver or the taker) then really feel into your body for what you would like. If the touch is for your partner (i.e. you are the giver or the allower), then pause and check in with your body to sense if you are truly willing to grant your partner's wishes. This exercise works with any form of touch so it is easy to do it in a non-sexual way with a friend too.

Practising each of these roles is a great way to explore how to notice what we want, what we're happy to do, how to communicate it, and what to do if things change. It also helps spotlight any unhelpful habits we have got into where we tend towards always playing one role (e.g. always being the giver) and what other roles might really work for us sexually.

CHAPTER 19

COMMUNICATION IS SEXY

No matter how much sex we have had or how dominant any societal sexpectation is, it is never good to assume you know what works for a partner. Different bodies experience the world differently and we need to explore what each individual finds pleasurable on any given day. Not all women's bodies work the same, nor do all men's. When we base our assumptions on what works for someone based on sexpectations, past history with them or other partners or what we ourselves like, no one wins.

Most people are self-referential. We are biased to think that everyone else experiences the world like we do and we find it difficult to grasp that whatever we like to do sexually may be repulsive to someone else. Similarly, whatever disgusts us sexually might be the most treasured, special and sexual experience for someone else. Most people mistake their sexual preferences for a universal rule book that should work for everyone. For example, one study found that people in long-term relationships only knew 60% of what their partner liked sexually and about 20% of what they didn't like (Byers, 2005). Moreover, because of the myth that a "good" partner should *know* what works, as if by telepathy, we rarely give ourselves the opportunity to correct this mistake through communication.

> *'I couldn't believe it when he told me he didn't actually like anal sex. I thought all guys wanted anal, because ... you know, porn ... so I put up with it. When I think back to the amount of times I could have saved myself the stress and had the sex I wanted!'* – **Tara**

No two people are the same, and every person has similarities and differences to each other. This holds true as much for sex as it does in other areas of life. Think about sexual similarities and differences like a Venn diagram of what you are up for now and what they are up for now. The place where each of you will find yourself able to be fully present and embodied will be in the overlap space. This will lead to you both having the sex you really want.

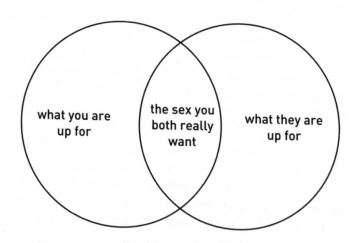

As such it's okay if we don't find all the same things arousing as our partner(s). However, it is important to remain respectful and actively strive to understand what works for our partner without judgement. For the interests we have outside the overlap, we can explore what other options are available to indulge them, depending on how important they feel to us as a couple and the agreements in our relationship.

In a monogamous relationship, a partner might be willing to role play some things with us or talk *as if* we're going to do something, even if they aren't interested in participating in real life. Similarly, a partner may have a genuine willingness to dabble or engage in part of what excites us, even if they are not too fussed about it themselves (i.e. they will put themselves in the giving or allowing role that we spoke about in the Wheel of Consent in the last chapter). However, it is important to acknowledge that things won't always work out – it is possible to have a lot of love and attraction for someone but no overlap in what you are into sexually.

'I just find it really hard to find someone with the full package. I want to be attracted to my partner, to be able to have intelligent conversations and share the same interests. It would be great if she wasn't a crazy person too! But I'm not sure I can give up my kinky side and I just haven't met anyone who has ticked all these boxes who would tolerate that in a relationship' – **John**

Most people are very sensitive with asking for what they want, giving and getting sexual feedback. We want to please our partners and "get it right". No one likes to feel rejected. So, although asking for what you want and giving feedback is a gift – it helps someone who wants to please you to do that most effectively – we need to be sensitive and skilful in how we communicate it, while still being truthful and respecting our boundaries. Below are some tips to help you develop sexy, skilful communication.

Giving Feedback

1. Be specific – feedback like "fine" or "good" will never get you closer to the touch that works for you. Instead, describe what is good or give it a rating.

   'I love the sensation of you nibbling on my thigh – that was really hot.'

   'I'm at a seven out of ten on my pain threshold.'

2. Be encouraging – where possible, focus on what you liked rather than what you didn't.

   'I liked it when you pulled my hair, could you try that again?'

3. Offer an alternative – instead of just saying "no" or "don't", offer an alternative if you can do so authentically.

   'I'd love to try this a little slower.'

4. Sandwich negative feedback – start with something encouraging and end with an alternative.

   'I love how much you love my breasts, but they are hurting now and we need to stop. Could you touch my belly instead?'

5. Be kind – try not to criticise or be judgemental, give them feedback in the way you'd like to receive it.

   'You are very enthusiastic! It's great and I'm wondering if we can take it a little slower.'

Asking for Feedback

1. Don't ask, 'Is this okay?' – "okay" is an unhelpful four-letter word when it comes to sex because who would really want the way we are touching someone to be just okay? The same can be said for the other four-letter words "fine" and "good".

2. Ask open questions – This will give you much more helpful information than a question that gives you a yes/no answer. *'What would make this feel even better?'*

3. Offer a choice – When you offer two alternatives (preferably while you are demonstrating the choices!) you help your partner make a more embodied choice. *'Would you like it harder or softer [faster/slower, here/there, etc.]?'*

4. Offer a scale – This will also give you richer information. *'Out of ten, how much did you like that?'*

Asking for What you Want

1. Be embodied — make sure you take the time to check in with your body to see if you are really into something, rather than asking out of habit or for another reason.

2. Be brave – lots of people fear embarrassment or rejection but all our desires are acceptable and communicating them will help you and your partner grow closer and have the sex you really want.

3. Use "if" statements – make requests that allow an easy no by giving your partner an out. *'If you have the energy, I'd love to try anal tonight.'*

4. Ask to show them – sometimes it's easier to show rather than tell. *'Can I give you a foot rub in the way I like my feet rubbed to show you?'*

5. Change your mind – follow where the sexual energy leads. Sometimes a no becomes a yes, and a yes becomes a no, so give yourself permission to communicate the updates as they happen.

6. Don't take it personally – There is nothing inherently shameful about any desire you have even if your partner is not into it. In fact, asking for what we want can help dissolve any shame or self-consciousness, even when our partner says no.

When Receiving a "No"

1. Don't take it personally – think about how the person has honoured themselves and be grateful that they made it easy for you to make things work for them.
2. Say thank you – a no is a gift that builds trust and allows for much better sex. The more we can trust a partner to say no, the more we can dare to ask for.
3. Don't give up – a no is a yes to something else, you just need to find it!
4. If it's not a clear yes, it's a no – it's better to be safe than sorry, so if there is any ambiguity, clarify it or err on the side of caution.

WHEN ACTIONS AND WORDS DON'T MATCH

It's great if we can get clear, verbal communication from our partners but this is an ideal that is rarely achieved in real life. Different partners have different levels of skilfulness with knowing what they want and comfort with communicating it. As such, it is useful to be observant and look for whether their verbal feedback matches the feedback you are picking up from their body and behaviours.

Out of respect for a partner, it is generally good practice to take them on face value and not second-guess their yes. However, if things don't add up, we need to protect our own comfort. Forging ahead when we have a suspicion our partner is not being genuine with their consent will only ever make for a fraught sexual experience.

Ambiguous or suspect communication can include:

- They seem to avoid giving an answer
- They say yes but seem distracted or disconnected
- They say yes but then avoid the interaction or cancel repeatedly
- They say things like "I don't mind" or "Do what you want" or "It's ok"
- They say yes but their body tells a different story such as they are leaning away, can't make eye contact or have gone unusually quiet
- They say they don't have any limits
- They say they liked everything but can't be specific
- They keep forgetting what you've said or what you've asked for

EXERCISE: CAMP COMMUNICATION

When was the last time you and your partner talked about what you have been doing together sexually and physically outside of the sexual experiences themselves? How would you bring it up if you did? Could you find some space to make this kind of sexual State of the Union a regular ritual in your relationship?

Practise asking for what you want – sit back to back or use text to create more of a safe space. When you are brave enough, you can do it sitting face to face and making eye contact. Take turns using the simple statement "I want you to..." or "I want to", and when you receive the desires of your partner, just say thank you.

For example:

Person A: *'I want to suck your toes.'*

Person B: *'Thank you'* … *'I want you to kiss my thighs.'*

Person A: *'Thank you'* … *'I want you to give me a lap dance.'*

Person B: *'Thank you'* … *'I want to go down on you in a cinema.'*

Practise saying no – using the same method as asking for what you want, when you receive the desires of your partner, practise saying no instead of, or in addition to, thank you. You can say a simple "thank you, no" or versions of it like "no, that's not my thing" but make sure it's a clear and direct statement.

For example:

Person A: *'I want to suck your toes.'*

Person B: *'Thank you but no, that's not my thing'* … *'I want you to kiss my thighs.'*

Person A: *'No, but thanks for sharing'* … *'I want you to give me a lap dance.'*

Person B: *'thank you, but no, I'm not into that today'* … *'I want to go down on you in a cinema.'*

EXPLORING YOUR EDGES

It is likely that at various times we will have mixed feelings about certain sexual experiences, requests and offers. This is true for most decisions we make in life and situations we find ourselves in. For example, there may be a part of us that really wants to meet a friend for coffee and another part that just wants to stay home on the couch. Using the presence and embodiment skills we have developed can help us unpack our ambivalence and be open to what is drawing us towards and pushing us away from something or someone with curiosity and openness.

It can be useful to explore the relative strength of each part of our response, and the reason for them. Maybe 60% of you would like to receive oral sex, but 40% of you feels uncomfortable about it because you haven't showered. You might then think about compromises or deals to help resolve the ambivalence satisfactorily – in this case, asking to take a shower might evaporate the 40% of "no"s.

Stepping over our consent is unkind to ourselves, it leaves us enjoying sex less than before, and it leaves the other person feeling disconnected from us at best, and at worst, terribly guilty if they realise we weren't really into it. At the same time, what works for us and what doesn't constantly evolves based on our experiences, new or changing relationships, and our own personal development. We will never know every single detail of exactly what makes us tick in the bedroom, and that's okay. Part of growth in any area is finding and playing at our edges.

Being open to experimenting with new and different things, both on our own and with a partner(s) can help us expand our self-knowledge and help us stay in touch with our changing needs. There's no way to fully know whether or not we'll like something unless we try it whilst making sure to stay connected to our embodied feedback.

Of course, we all have boundaries that we know we don't want to go beyond. At the same time, it's also exciting to give ourselves permission to explore things in a gradual, safe and controlled way. For example, if having a threesome has never really been your thing, but there's nothing about it that feels unsafe to you, then that may be an edge that you can explore. You might like to start out by trying it on for size first by fantasising about it or talking dirty about it with a partner, without actually doing it.

EXERCISE: AMBIVALENCE PIE

Go back to a recent sexual opportunity or experience that you felt some ambivalence about. Map out your different feelings on a pie chart and give each slice a relative percentage. Write the reasons you think that part of you felt that way, and part of you felt another and part of you a third and so on.

Thinking back to the decision you made around that situation, did you acknowledge all these parts? How could you make a more balanced and embodied choice in the future?

PART 3: SUMMARY AND EXERCISES

You are in a far better place to be a skilful lover and to receive the touch you want when you are out of your head, connected to and tracking the sensations in your body, and able to communicate to your partner what you want as well as respond to them.

However, gaining skilfulness in being present and embodied takes practice. As such we recommend beginning a thirty-day challenge. Whether you decide to engage in sexual self-touch or sexual activity with a partner, put aside fifteen to thirty minutes each day for thirty days. Set a timer with a gentle bell at the end so you can get absorbed in your experience without clock-watching.

Use one of the embodiment practices I have suggested (or your own relaxation strategy) to calm your mind and get into your body. Then, listen to your body for what it wants that day.

You may find that you just want to lie down with your hands laying on top of your pelvis. You may want to be touched on the non-genital areas of your body. You may discover that you want a full orgasmic experience. There is no right or wrong and no activity you have to achieve, so long as you are aware of and listening to your body's signals. Whatever you feel like your body needs that day is perfect.

Watch also for any thoughts and excuses that come up for you. We often don't prioritise our sex life and put ourselves last on the list of where we spend our time and energy. Try to work through whatever blocks come up for you so that you can give yourself the time and energy you deserve.

CONCLUSION

AS IN SEX, SO IN LIFE

It isn't a big stretch to think back over what you have read and realise that we aren't just talking about sex here. We have expectations and culturally endorsed messages for just about everything we experience in life and no one is totally unbiased as a result. Therefore, just as it can be illuminating to explore the sexpectations behind any aspects of sex that aren't working for you, it can also be transformational too to unpick the expectations you have around other areas of your life. What do you believe? How did you come to adopt those beliefs? Where do those beliefs hold you back?

Similarly, your body is your constant companion throughout your life and will be incessantly offering you information in the form of sensory and emotional data, should you choose to pay attention to it. It is amazing what you can learn about yourself and what works for you in so many aspects of life – with food, with friends, at work, in how you exercise, etc. – if you just pay attention!

Awareness and respect of our bodies' boundaries can have a profound impact on our self-esteem, our experience of the world, and our relationships. When it comes to noticing and communicating our desires and our limits, it's about so much more than sex – it's about the greater task of living and negotiating our way in the world.

Embodied consent is about honouring our sense of being in the world and our bodies' boundaries. As Brene Brown said, "daring to set boundaries is about having the courage to love ourselves, even when we risk disappointing others" (2015). Whether we are saying no to staying back late at work; saying no to sharing our dessert or saying no to sex we aren't into, we owe it to ourselves to act lovingly towards ourselves in this way.

Our boundaries conversely allow us to be truly intimate with others – saying no to someone you care about can be a vulnerable and revealing act. Boundaries also allow us to give to others wholeheartedly – without resentment or disengagement. There is never a true yes when we don't have the ability to say no, and it is so much better for everyone involved when we spend our time doing things we are truly into.

So, next time you find yourself complaining or resentful, bitter or angry about something or someone, stop. Ask yourself which of your boundaries have been crossed here? What have you needed to say no to? How could you be more self-protective and truthful so you don't allow yourself to be in situations that make you feel like this again? Your feelings are your body's way of communicating about what you need, so don't waste your energy focusing on things that "should" be different in your situation, or what someone else "shouldn't" have done. You can only control you.

Making it our mission to develop skilfulness in recognising our embodied boundaries and expressing our desires and limits is a gift to ourselves and anyone we interact with. Like any skill, it gets better with practice and I personally can't think of any more enjoyable practice ground than whilst having sex!

Reading through this book, and doing the exercises, you've had the chance to learn and discover how your sexpectations have developed and why. You may have had your sexual beliefs challenged, your regular way of thinking altered. With ongoing awareness and practice checking in with your body, being present during sex and communicating what works for you during partnered sex, you may find that what you want out of sex changes. Likewise, applying these skills to your broader life may help you understand more about what you truly want in life as well.

Use this information to empower yourself to try something new, to not just stretch those boundaries you have for yourself, but create new boundaries. Empower yourself to live the life that *you* want to live, based on your embodied wants and needs. Communicate your true self with those around you, and in doing so surround yourself with people who truly know, respect and love you.

Reading through this book will help you understand your boundaries, so dip back into it at any time you need a refresher. You can also share it with a friend or partner who you think could benefit from having their sexpectations challenged. However, only putting this advice into action will help you truly connect with your embodied desires. As such, we've reached the point where we encourage you to stop reading, feel into your body and what you truly need right now … and go for it!

ACKNOWLEDGEMENTS

We want to thank all the people at Trigger Publishing as well as all the people in our own lives who helped make this book happen. Whether you were an active participant or someone who just gave us the space to hermit ourselves away to write most weekends – we appreciate it!

We also want to acknowledge and thank all the generous people who have shared their experiences with us, thereby allowing readers to connect with their stories as if they were their own.

REFERENCES

Abma, J. C. and Martinex, G. M. (2017). Sexual Activity and Contraceptive Use Among Teenagers in the United States. *National Health Stat Report*, (104), pp. 1–23.

Acevedo, B. P. and Aron, A. (2009). Does a long-term relationship kill romantic love? *Review of General Psychology*, 13, pp. 59–65.

Acevedo, B. P., Aron, A., Fisher, H. E. and Brown L. L. (2012). Neural correlates of long-term intense romantic love. *Social Cognitive and Affective Neuroscience*, 7(2), pp. 145–159.

Ålgars, M., Santtila, P., Jern P., Johansson, A., Westerlund, M. and Sandnabba, N.K. (2011). Sexual body image and its correlates: A population-based study of Finnish women and men. *International Journal of Sexual Health*, 23(1), pp. 26–34.

Ambrosino, B. (2019). Are we set for a new sexual revolution? [Online] BBC Future. Available at: https://www.bbc.com/

future/article/20190702-are-we-set-for-a-new-sexual-revolution [Accessed 24.01.2020]

Anapol, D. (2010). *Polyamory in the 21st Century*. Landham, MD: Rowman & Littlefield Publishing.

Archer, J. and Lloyd, B. (2014). *Sex and Gender*. Cambridge: Cambridge University Press.

Armstrong, E. A., England, P. and Fogarty, A. C. K. (2012). Accounting for Women's Orgasm and Sexual Enjoyment in College Hook-ups and Relationships. *American Sociological Review*, 77(3), pp. 435–462.

Bancroft, J., Loftus, J. and Long, S. J. (2003). Distress About Sex: A National Survey of Women in Heterosexual Relationships. *Archives of Sexual Behaviour,* 32, pp. 193–208.

Baranowski, A. M. and Hecht, H. (2015). Gender Differences and Similarities in Receptivity to Sexual Invitations: Effects of Location and Risk Perception. *Archives of Sexual Behaviour,* (8), pp. 2257–2265.

Basson, R. (2000). The Female Sexual Response Revisited. *Journal SOGC,* 22(5), pp. 378–382.

Baumeister, R. F., Catanese, K. and Vohs, K. (2001). Is There a Gender Difference in Strength of Sex Drive? Theoretical Views, Conceptual Distinctions, and a Review of Relevant Evidence. *Personality and Social Psychology Review,* 5(3), pp. 242–273.

Baumeister, R. F. (2000). Gender differences in erotic plasticity: the female sex drive as socially flexible and responsive. *Psychological Bulletin*, 126(3), pp. 347–374.

Beck, J., Bozman, A. and Qualtrough, T. (1991). The Experience of Sexual Desire: Psychological correlates in a college sample. *Journal of Sex Research*, 28(3), pp. 443–456.

Bellah, R. N., Madsen, R., Sullivan, W. M., Swidler, A. and Tipton, S. M. (1985). *Habits of the Heart: Individualism and Commitment in American Life*. New York: Harper & Row.

Bendixen, M., Kennair, L. and Grøntvedt, T. (2018). Forgiving the unforgivable: Couples' forgiveness and expected forgiveness of emotional and sexual infidelity from an error management theory perspective. *Evolutionary Behavioural Sciences*, 12(4), pp. 322–335.

Berman, L., Berman, J., Miles, M., Pollets, D. and Powell, J. A. (2003). Genital self-image as a component of sexual health: Relationship between genital self-image, female sexual function, and quality of life measures. *Journal of Sex & Marital Therapy*, 29, pp. 11–21.

Birkhead, T. (2000). *Promiscuity: An evolutionary history of sperm competition*. Cambridge, Mass.: Harvard University Press.

Birnbaum, G. E. and Finkel, E. J. (2015). The magnetism that holds us together: Sexuality and relationship maintenance across relationship development. *Current Opinion in Psychology*, 1, pp. 29–33.

Bischmann, A., Richardson, C., O'Leary, J., Gullickson, M., Davidson, M. and Gervais, S. (2017). Age and Experience of First Exposure to Pornography: Relations to Masculine Norms. Poster Session, Thursday, Aug. 3 August, 2017, 11 1-11:50 a.m. EDT, Halls D and E, Level 2, Walter E. Washington Convention Center, 801 Mount Vernon Pl., N.W., Washington, D.C.

Blair, K. and Pukall, C. (2014). Can less be more? Comparing duration vs. frequency of sexual encounters in same-sex and mixed-sex relationships. *The Canadian Journal of Human Sexuality*, 23(2), pp. 123-136.

Blume, J. (1975). *Forever: A Novel*. Scarsdale, NY: Bradbury Press.

Blumstein, P. and Schwartz, P. (1983). *American Couples: Money, Work, Sex*. New York: William Morrow.

Bogart, L. M., Cecil, H., Wagstaff, D. A., Pinkerton, S. D. and Abramson, P. R. (2000). Is it "Sex"?: college students' interpretations of sexual behaviour terminology. *Journal of Sex Research*. 37, pp. 108–116.

Bogle, K. (2007). The Shift from Dating to Hooking Up in College: What Scholars Have Missed. *Sociology Compass*, 1(2), pp. 775–788.

Braun, V. (2005). In Search of (Better) Sexual Pleasure: Female Genital 'Cosmetic' Surgery. *Sexualities*, 8(4), pp. 407–424.

Brody, S. (2010). The Relative Health Benefits of Different Sexual Activities. *The Journal of Sexual Medicine*, 7(4), pp. 1336–1361.

Brody, S. and Krüger, T. (2006). The post-orgasmic prolactin increase following intercourse is greater than following masturbation and suggests greater satiety. *Biological Psychology*, 71(3), pp. 312–315.

Brown, B. (2015). *Rising Strong.* London: Vermilion.

Byers, E. (2005). Relationship satisfaction and sexual satisfaction: A longitudinal study of individuals in long-term relationships. *Journal of Sex Research*, 42(2), pp. 113–118.

Carpenter, C. J. and McEwan B. (2016). The players of micro-dating: individual and gender differences in goal orientations toward mirco-dating apps. *First Monday: Peer-Reviewed Journal on the Internet, Vol.* 21, (No. 5).

Carpenter, L. M. (2005). *Virginity Lost: An Intimate Portrait of First Sexual Experiences.* New York: New York University Press.

Carson, C. and Gunn, K. (2006). Premature ejaculation: definition and prevalence. *International Journal of Impotence Research.* Sep–Oct, *18*(1), pp. Suppl 1: S5–13.

Carswell, K. L. and Finkel, E. J. (2018). Can you get the magic back? The moderating effect of passion decay beliefs on relationship commitment. *Journal of Personality and Social Psychology*, 115, pp. 1002–1032.

Chaney, M.P., (2008). Muscle dysmorphia, self-esteem, and loneliness among gay and bisexual men. *International Journal of Men's Health*, 7(2), p.157.

Charnetski, C. J. and Brennan, F. X. (2004). Sexual frequency and salivary immunoglobulin A (IgA). *Psychology Report*, 94 (3 Pt 1), pp. 839–844.

Cherlin, A. J. (2004). The Deinstitutionalisation of Marriage. *Journal of Marriage and Family*, 66, pp. 848–862.

Christopher, F.S. and Sprecher, S. (2000). Sexuality in Marriage, Dating, and Other Relationships: A Decade Review. *Journal of Marriage and Family*, 62, pp. 999–1017.

Chrystal, P. (2016). *In Bed with the Ancient Greeks: Sex & Sexuality in Ancient Greece*, p. 25. Stroud, UK: Amberley Publishing.

Collins, R. L., Martino, S. C., Elliott, M. N. and Miu, A. (2011). Relationships Between Adolescent Sexual Outcomes and Exposure to Sex in Media: Robustness to Propensity-Based Analysis. *Developmental Psychology*, 47(2), pp. 585–591.

Connelly, C. (2018). *Off limits*. Sydney: Harlequin, Mills & Boon.

Connelly, D. (2017). Three decades of Viagra, *The Pharmaceutical Journal*, 298, (No 7901).

Cooke, R. (2010). Fifty years of the pill. Available at: https://www.theguardian.com/society/2010/jun/06/rachel-cooke-fifty-years-the-pill-oral-contraceptive. [Accessed:24.01.2020]

Cranney, S. (2015). Internet pornography use and sexual body image in a Dutch sample. *International Journal of Sexual Health*, 27(3), pp. 316–323.

Critelli, J. W. and Bivona, J. M. (2008). Women's Erotic Rape Fantasies: An Evaluation of Theory and Research, *The Journal of Sex Research*, 45(1), pp. 57–70.

Dabbs, J. M. and Mohammed, S. (1992). Male and female salivary testosterone concentrations before and after sexual activity, *Physiology & Behaviour*, 52(1), pp. 195–197.

Davidson, J. (2001). Dover, Foucault And Greek Homosexuality: Penetration And The Truth Of Sex. The Use Of Greeks. *Past & Present*, 170(1), pp. 3–51.

de Cuypere, G., T'Sjoen, G., Beerten, R., Selvaggi, G., De Sutter, P., Hoebeke, P., Monstrey, S., Vansteenwegen, A. and Rubens, R. (2005). Sexual and Physical Health After Sex Reassignment Surgery. *Archives of Sexual Behaviour*, 34(6), pp. 679–690.

de Prorok, Count B. (1935). *In Quest of Lost Worlds*. NY: E.P. Dutton.

DePaulo, B. (2011). *Singlism: What it is, why it matters and how to stop it.* Charleston, NC: DoubleDoor Books.

Derrida, J. (1968). Plato's Pharmacy. Translated by B.Johnson (ed). Dissemination. Chicago.IL: University of Chicago Press. pp. 61–171 (1981).

Diamond, J. (1997). *Guns, Germs and Steel*. New York: W.W. Norton.

Diamond, L. (2009). *Sexual fluidity*. Cambridge, Mass.: Harvard University Press.

Diamond, L. M. (2012). The Desire Disorder in Research on Sexual Orientation in Women: Contributions of Dynamical Systems Theory. *Archives of Sexual Behaviour*, 41, pp. 73–83.

Dimitropoulou, P., Lophatananon, A., Easton, D., Pocock, R., Dearnaley, D.P., Guy, M., Edwards, S., O'Brien, L., Hall, A., Wilkinson, R., Eeles, R. and Muir, K.R. (2009). Sexual activity and prostate cancer risk in men diagnosed at a younger age. *BJU International*, 103(2), pp. 178–185.

Dion, K., Berscheid, E. and Walster, E. (1972). What is beautiful is good. *Journal of Personality and Social Psychology*, 24(3), pp. 285–290.

Doidge, N. (2007). *The Brain that Changes Itself*. New York: Viking.

Dutton, D. and Aron, A. (1974). Some evidence for heightened sexual attraction under conditions of high anxiety. *Journal of Personality and Social Psychology*, 30(4), pp. 510–517.

Dworkin, S. L. and O'Sullivan, L. (2005). Actual versus desired initiation patterns among a sample of college men:

tapping disjuncture within traditional male sexual scripts. *Journal of Sex Research.* 42(2), pp. 150–158.

Dynes, W. R. and Donaldson, S. (1992). *Homosexuality in the Ancient World.* London: Taylor and Francis.

Ellis, H. (1946). *Psychology of Sex.* New York: Emerson Books.

Evans-Pritchard, E. (1971). *The Azande.* Oxford: Clarendon Press.

Faderman, L. (1981). *Surpassing the Love of Men: Romantic Friendship and Love Between Women from the Renaissance to the Present.* New York: Quill.

Fakhry, A. (1973). *Siwa Oasis.* Cairo: The American University in Cairo Press.

Feldman, H. A., et al. (1998). Low Dehydroepiandrosterone Sulphate and Heart Disease in Middle-Aged Men: Cross-sectional Results from the Massachusetts Male Aging Study. *Annals of Epidemiology*, 8(4), pp. 217–228.

Fisher, H. (2016). *Anatomy Of Love: A Natural History of Mating, Marriage, and Why We Stray.* New York: W. W. Norton & Company.

Fisher, T. D., Moore, Z. T. and Pittenger, M. (2012). Sex on the brain? An examination of frequency of sexual cognitions as a function of gender, erotophilia, and social desirability. *Journal of Sex Research,* 29, pp. 69–77.

Fone, B.R.S. (2000). *Homophobia: A History*. New York: Metropolitan Books.

Frederick, D. A. and Essayli, J.H. (2016). Male Body Image: The Roles of Sexual Orientation and Body Mass Index Across Five National U.S. Studies. *Psychology of Men & Masculinity*, 17(4), pp. 336–351.

Freitas, D. (2013). *The End of Sex: How Hook-up Culture is Leaving a Generation Unhappy, Sexually Unfulfilled, and Confused About Intimacy*. New York: Basic Books.

Freud, S. (1951). Letter to an American Mother. *American Journal of Psychiatry*, 107(10), pp. 786–787.

Friedman, H., and Martin, L. (2011). *The Longevity Project: Surprising Discoveries for Health and Long Life from the Landmark Eight-Decade Study*. New York: Hudson Street Press.

Gagnon, J. H. (1973). Scripts and the coordination of sexual conduct. *Nebraska Symposium on Motivation*. University of Nebraska Press, pp. 27–59.

Gagnon, J. H. and Parker, R. G. (1995). *Conceiving sexuality: Approaches to sex research in a postmodern world*. New York: Routledge.

Gahran, A. (2017). *Stepping off the Relationship Escalator: Uncommon Love and life*. Boulder, CO: Off the Escalator Enterprises, LLC.

Garcia, J. R. and Reiber, C. (2008). Hook-up behaviour: A biopsychosocial perspective. *Journal of Social, Evolutionary, and Cultural Psychology,* 2(4), pp. 192–208.

Garcia, J. R., Reiber, C., Massey, S. G. and Merriwether, A. M., (2013). Sexual Hook-up Culture. *Review of General Psychology,* 16(2), pp. 161–176.

Gavey, N., McPhillips, K. and Braun, V. (1999). Interruptus Coitus: Heterosexuals Accounting for Intercourse. *Sexualities,* 2. pp. 35–68.

Gerressu, M., Mercer, C.H., Graham, C.A., Wellings, K. and Johnson, A.M. (2007). Prevalence of Masturbation and Associated Factors in a British National Probability Survey. *Archives of Sexual Behaviour,* 37(2) pp. 266–278.

Gibbs, N. (2010). The Pill at 50: Sex, Freedom and Paradox. Available at: http://content.time.com/time/magazine/article/0,9171,1983884-1,00.html [Accessed on 24.01.2020]

Giles, G. G., Severi, G., English, D. R., McCredie, M. R. E., Borland, R., Boyle, P. and Hopper, J. L. (2003). Sexual factors and prostate cancer. *BJU International,* 92, pp. 211–216.

Gill, R. (2003). From sexual objectification to sexual subjectification: The resexualisation of women's bodies in the media. *Feminist Media Studies,* 3, pp. 100–106.

Glendon, M. A. (1989). *The transformation of family law: State, law, and family in the United States and Western Europe*. Chicago: University of Chicago Press.

Gordon, D., Porter, A., Regnerus, M., Ryngaert, J. and Sarangaya, L. (2014). Relationships in America Survey. *Relationships in America*. Available at: http://relationshipsinamerica.com/ [Accessed on 24.01.2020]

Gottman, J. and Silver, N. (2000). *The Seven Principles for Making Marriage Work: A Practical Guide from the Country's Foremost Relationship Expert*. New York: Harmony Books.

Haake, P., Krueger, T. H., Goebel, M. U., Heberling, K. M., Hartmann, U. and Schedlowski, M. (2004). Effects of sexual arousal on lymphocyte subset circulation and cytokine production in man. *Neuroimmunomodulation*, 11(5), pp. 293–298.

Hald, G., Malmuth, N., and Yuen, C. (2010). Pornography and Attitudes Supporting Violence Against Women: Revisiting the Relationship on Non-Experimental Studies, *Aggressive Behaviour*, 36, pp. 1065–1086.

Hall, S.A., Shackelton, R., Rosen, R.C., Araujo, A.B. (2010). Sexual Activity, Erectile Dysfunction, and Incident Cardiovascular Events. *American Journal of Cardiology*, 105(2), pp. 192–197.

Hornblower, S., ed., Spawforth, A., ed. and Eidinow, E., ed. (2012). *Oxford Classical Dictionary*, "homosexuality", pp. 720–723.

Harvey, K. (2018). Getting down and medieval: the sex lives of the Middle Ages. Available at: https://aeon.co/essays/getting-down-and-medieval-the-sex-lives-of-the-middle-ages [Accessed on 24.01.2020]

Heer, D. M., Grossbard-Shechtman, A. (1981). The Impact of the Female Marriage Squeeze and the Contraceptive Revolution on Sex Roles and the Women's Liberation Movement in the United States, 1960 to 1975. *Journal of Marriage and the Family*, 43(1), pp. 49–65.

Heiman, J. R., Long, J. S., Smith, S. N., Fisher, W. A., Sand, M. S. and Rosen, R. C. (2011). Sexual satisfaction and relationship happiness in midlife and older couples in five countries. *Archives of Sexual Behaviour*, 40(4), pp. 741–753.

Heldman, C. and Wade, L. (2010). Hook-Up Culture: Setting a New Research Agenda. *Sexuality Research and Social Policy,* 7(4), pp. 323–333.

Herbenick, D., Bowling, J., Fu, T., Dodge, B., Guerra-Reyes, L. and Sanders, S. (2017). Sexual diversity in the United States: Results from a nationally representative probability sample of adult women and men. [Online] *PLOS ONE*, 12(7). Available at: https://doi.org/10.1371/journal.pone.0181198

Herbenick, D., Reece, M., Schick, V., Sanders, S. A., Dodge, B., and Fortenberry, J. D. (2010). Sexual behaviour in the United States: Results from a national probability sample of men and women ages 14–94. *The Journal of Sexual Medicine* 7, pp. 255–265.

Hess, J., Rossi Neto, R., Panic, L., Rübben, H. and Senf, W. (2014). Satisfaction with male-to-female gender reassignment surgery. *Deutsches Arzteblatt international*, 111(47), pp. 795–801.

Hickman, S.E. and Muehlenhard, C.L. (1999). By the Semi-mystical Appearance of a Condom: How Young Women and Men Communicate Sexual Consent in Heterosexual Situations, *The Journal of Sex Research*, 36, pp. 258–272.

Hinsliff, G. (2015). Consent is not enough: if you want a sexual partner, look for enthusiasm. Available at: https://www.theguardian.com/commentisfree/2015/jan/29/rape-consent-sexual-partner-enthusiasm [Accessed on 24.01.2020]

Hogenboom, M. (2015). Are there any homosexual animals? [Online] BBC Earth. Available at: http://www.bbc.com/earth/story/20150206-are-there-any-homosexual-animals [Accessed on 24.01.2020]

Huang, H. (2018). Cherry Picking: Virginity Loss Definitions Among Gay and Straight Cisgender Men, *Journal of Homosexuality*, 65(6), pp. 727–740.

Hunter Murray, S. (2019). *Not Always in the Mood: The New Science of Men, Sex, and Relationships*. Landham, MD: Rowman & Littlefield Publishing.

Jackson, S. (2006). Gender, sexuality and heterosexuality: the complexity (and limits) of heteronormativity. *Feminist Theory* 7, pp. 105–121.

Jennings, R. (2007). *A Lesbian History of Britain*. Santa Barabara, CA: Greenwood World Publishing.

Joel, D., Berman, D., Tavor, I., Wexler, N., Gaber, O., Stein, Y., Shefi, N., Pool, J., Urchs, S., Margulies, D. S., Liem, F., Hänggi, J., Jäncke, L. and Assaf, Y., (2015). Sex beyond the genitalia: The human brain mosaic. *Proceedings of the National Academy of Sciences*, 112(50).

Kaplan, H. S. (1979). Hypoactive sexual desire. *Journal of Sex & Marital Therapy*, 3, pp. 3–9.

Katz, J. (1995). *Gay and American History: Lesbians and Gay Men in the United States*. New York: Thomas Crowell.

Kellerman, J., Lewis, J. and Laird, J. (1989). Looking and loving: The effects of mutual gaze on feelings of romantic love. *Journal of Research in Personality*, 23, pp. 145–161.

King, R. (1997). *Good Loving, Great Sex*. Sydney: Random House.

Kinsey, A. C. (1948). *Sexual Behaviour in the Human Male*. Philadelphia: W. B. Saunders.

Kontula, O. and Haavio-Mannila, E. (2003). Masturbation in a Generational Perspective. *Journal of Psychology & Human Sexuality*, 14(2–3), pp. 49–83.

Kruger, D., Fisher, M., Edelstein, R., Chopik, W., Fitzgerald, C. and Strout, S. (2013). Was that cheating?

Perceptions vary by sex, attachment anxiety and behaviour. *Evolutionary Psychology*, 11(1), pp. 159–171.

Kühn, S. and Gallinat, J. (2014). Brain Structure and Functional Connectivity Associated With Pornography Consumption. *JAMA Psychiatry*, 71(7), pp. 827–834.

Kunkel, D., Eyal, K., Finnerty, K., Biely, E. and Donnerstein, E., (2005). *Sex on TV 2005: A Kaiser Family Foundation Report*. Menlo Park, CA: Henry J. Kaiser Family Foundation.

Kushner, D. (2019). *The Players Ball: A Genius, a Con Man, and the Secret History of the Internet's Rise*. Sydney: Simon & Schuster.

Lambert, R. (1984). *Beloved and God: The Story of Hadrian and Antinious*. London. George Weidenfeld & Nicolson.

Langer, G., Arnedt, C. and Sussman, D. (2004). The American Sex Survey: A Peek Beneath the Sheets. Retrieved from: http://abcnews.go.com/images/Politics/959a1AmericanSexSurvey.pdf [Accessed on 1st March 2020.]

Laumann, E.O., Ellingson, S., Mahay, J., Paik, A. and Youm, Y. (2004). *The Sexual Organization of the City*. Chicago: The University of Chicago Press.

Leitzmann, M.F., Platz, E.A., Stampfer, M.J., Willett, W.C., Giovannucci, E. (2004). Ejaculation Frequency and Subsequent Risk of Prostate Cancer. *JAMA, 291*(13), pp. 1578–1586.

Levine, E.C., Herbenick, D., Martinez, O., Fu, T.C., and Dodge, B. (2018). Open Relationships, Non-consensual Nonmonogamy, and Monogamy Among U.S. Adults: Findings from the 2012 National Survey of Sexual Health and Behaviour. *Archives of Sexual Behaviour,* 47 (5), pp. 1439–1450.

Levine, SB. (1987). More on the nature of sexual desire. *Journal of Sex & Marital Therapy,* 13, pp. 35–44.

Liao, L.M., Creighton, S.M., (2007). Requests for cosmetic genitoplasty: How should healthcare providers respond? *British Medical Journal, 334* (7603), pp. 1090–1092.

Lieberman, H. (2017). *Buzz: The Stimulating History of the Sex Toy.* New York: Pegasus Books.

Lily, Z. (2014). How to ace sex: Why enthusiastic consent doesn't cut it. [Online] The Standford Daily. Available at: https://www.stanforddaily.com/2014/11/04/how-to-ace-sex-why-enthusiastic-consent-doesnt-cut-it/_[Accessed on 24.01.2020]

Lloyd, E. (2006). *The Case of the Female Orgasm: Bias in the Science of Evolution.* Cambridge, Mass.: Harvard University Press.

Luff, T., Hoffman, K. and Berntson, M. (2016). Hooking Up and Dating are Two Sides of a Coin. *Contexts,* 15(1), pp. 76–77.

MacNeil, K. (2018). The Story of Viagra, the Little Blue Pill That Changed Sex Forever. [Online] VICE.com Available at: https://www.vice.com/en_au/article/mbxgnx/

the-story-of-viagra-the-little-blue-pill-that-changed-sex-forever. [Accessed on 24.01.2020]

Maines, R (1999). *The Technology of Orgasm: "Hysteria", the Vibrator, and Women's Sexual Satisfaction*. Baltimore, MD: Johns Hopkins University Press.

Manning, J. (2006). The Impact Internet Pornography on Marriage and the Family: A Review of the Research. *Sexual Addiction and Compulsivity*, 13, pp. 131–165.

Mark, K.P. (2012). The relative impact of individual sexual desire and couple desire discrepancy on satisfaction in heterosexual couples. *Sexual and Relationship Therapy*, 27(2), pp. 133–146.

Mark, W. (2013). Web porn: Just how much is there? [Online] BBC News. Available at: https://www.bbc.com/news/technology-23030090 [Accessed on 24.01.2020]

Marks, L. V., (2001). *Sexual Chemistry: A History of the Contraceptive Pill*. New Haven, CT: Yale University Press.

Masters, N. T., Casey, E., Wells, E. A., Morrison, D. M. (2013). Sexual scripts among young heterosexually active men and women: continuity and change. *Journal of Sex Research*, 50(5), pp. 409–420.

Masters, W. H., Johnson, V. E. (1970). *Human sexual inadequacy*. Boston, MA: Little, Brown.

May, E. (2010). *America and the Pill: A History of Promise, Peril and Liberation*. New York: Basic Books.

McGill, C.M. and Collins, J.C., (2014). Bottom identity: Matters of learning and development. SFERC 2014, p.8.

Medley-Rath, S. R. (2007). "Am I Still A Virgin?": What counts as sex in 20 years of *Seventeen*. *Sex. Cult.* 11, pp. 24–38.

Mendos, R.L. (2019). State-sponsored Homophobia. Geneva. ILGA, p.15.

Mercer, C. H., et al. (2013). Changes in sexual attitudes and lifestyles in Britain through the life course and over time: findings from the National Surveys of Sexual Attitudes and Lifestyles (Natsal). *Lancet,* 382 (9907), pp. 1757–1856.

Meston, C. and Buss, D. (2007). Why humans have sex. *Archives of Sexual Behaviour,* 36, pp. 477–507.

Meston, C. M., and Frohlich, P. F. (2003). Love at First Fright: Partner Salience Moderates Roller-Coaster-Induced Excitation Transfer. *Archives of Sexual Behaviour,* 32(6), pp. 537–544.

Miller, S. A. and Byers, E. S. (2004). Actual and desired duration of foreplay and intercourse: discordance and misperceptions within heterosexual couples. *Journal of Sex Research,* 41, pp. 301–309.

Mitchell, K. J., Ybarra, M. L., Korchmaros, J. D., Kosciw, J. G. (2014). Accessing sexual health information online: use, motivations and consequences for youth with different sexual orientations. *Health Education Research,* 29(1), pp. 147–157.

Mitchell, K. R., Geary, R., Graham, C. A., Datta, J., Wellings, K., Sonnenberg, P., Field, N., Nunns, D., Bancroft, J., Jones, K. G., Johnson, A. M., Mercer, C. H. (2017). Painful sex (dyspareunia) in women: prevalence and associated factors in a British population probability survey. *BJOG*, 124(11), pp. 1689–1697.

Mitricheva, E., Kimura, R., Logothetis, N. K., Noori, H. R. (2019). Neural substrates of sexual arousal are not sex dependent. *Proceedings of the National Academy of Sciences*, 116(31), pp. 15671–15676.

Montemurro, B. (2014). *Increasing our Understanding of Women's Sexuality: Deserving Desire: Women's Stories of Sexual Evolution*. New Jersey: Rutgers University Press.

Mowlabocus, S., Harbottle, J. and Witzel, C. (2013). Porn laid bare: Gay men, pornography and bareback sex. *Sexualities*, 16(5–6), pp. 523–547.

Mullinax, M., Herbenick, D., Schick, V., Sanders, S.A. and Reece, M. (2015). In their own words: a qualitative content analysis of women's and men's preferences for women's genitals. *Sex Education*, 15(4), pp. 421–436.

Murray, D. (2017). The consequence of this new sexual counter-revolution? No sex at all. [Online] The Spectator. Available at: https://www.spectator.co.uk/2017/11/the-consequence-of-this-new-sexual-counter-revolution-no-sex-at-all/ [Accessed on 24.01.2020]

Nagoski, E. (2015). *Come as you are: The surprising new science that will transform your sex life.* New York: Simon & Schuster.

Nakamura, J., Csikszentmihályi, M. (2001). Flow Theory and Research. In C. R. Snyder Erik Wright, and Shane J. Lopez (ed.). *Handbook of Positive Psychology.* Oxford: Oxford University Press.

Nast, C. (2019). Anal Sex: Safety, How tos, Tips, and More. [Online] *Teen Vogue* Available at: https://www.teenvogue.com/story/anal-sex-what-you-need-to-know [Accessed on 24.01.2020]

Naumann, E. (2004). *Love at first sight: The stories and science behind instant attraction.* Illinois: Sourcebooks, Inc..

Neill, J. (2011). *The Origins and Role of Same-Sex Relations in Human Societies.* Jefferson, NC: McFarland & Company.

Nicolson, P. and Burr, J. (2003). What is "normal" about women's (hetero)sexual desire and orgasm?: A report of an in-depth interview study. *Social Science Medical,* 57, pp. 1735–1745.

Norton, R (1998). *My Dear Boy: Gay Love Letters through the Centuries.* San Francisco: Leyland Publications.

Nussbaum, M. (1999). *Sex and Social Justice.* Oxford: Oxford University Press.

O'Donohue, W. and Plaud, J. J. (1991). The long-term habituation of sexual arousal in the human male. *Journal of Behaviour Therapy and Experimental Psychiatry,* 22(2), pp. 87–96.

O'Leary, D., Acevedo, B. P., Aron, A., Huddy, L. and Mashek, D. (2011). Is Long-Term Love More Than A Rare Phenomenon? If So, What Are Its Correlates? *Social Psychological and Personality Science,* 3(2), pp. 241–249.

Parish, William L., Luo, Ye., Stolzenberg, R., Laumann, E. O., Farrer, G. and Pan, S. (2007). Sexual Practices and Sexual Satisfaction: A Population Based Study of Chinese Urban Adults. *Archives of Sexual Behaviour,* 36, pp. 5–20.

Pascoe, C.J. (2012). *Dude, You're a Fag: Masculinity and Sexuality in High School.* Berkeley: University of California Press.

Patten, E. and Parker, K. (2012). A Gender Reversal On Career Aspirations: Young Women Now Top Young Men in Valuing a High-Paying Career. [Online] Pew Research Center. Available at: https://www.pewsocialtrends. org/2012/04/19/a-gender-reversal-on-career-aspirations/ [Accessed on 24.01.2020]

Paul, P. (2010). The cost of growing up with porn. [Online] Washington Post. Available at: http://www. washingtonpost.com/wp-dyn/content/article/2010/03/05/ AR2010030501552.html [Accessed on 24.01.2020]

Pederson, W. and Blekesaune, M. (2003). Sexual Satisfaction in Young Adulthood: Cohabitation, Committed Dating or Unattached Life? *Acta Sociologica,* 46, pp. 179–193.

Perel, E. (2017). Quoted in: **Walden, C.** Why putting sex on your 'to-do' list can save your marriage. [Online]

National Post. Available at: https://nationalpost.com/
health/why-putting-sex-on-your-to-do-list-can-actually-save-
your-marriage [Accessed on 24.01.2020]

Pertot, S. (2007). *When your Sex Drives Don't Match.* London:
Da Capo Lifelong Books.

Pham, J. (2016). The Limits of Heteronormative Sexual
Scripting: College Student Development of Individual
Sexual Scripts and Descriptions of Lesbian Sexual
Behaviour. *Frontiers in Sociology*, 1.

Plato. (1925). *Plato in Twelve Volumes, Vol. 9*, translated by
Harold N. Fowler. Cambridge, MA: Harvard University
Press; London: William Heinemann Ltd.

Popenoe, D. (1996). *Life without father: Compelling new evidence
that fatherhood and marriage are indispensable for the good of children
and society.* New York: Martin Kessler Books.

Potts, A. (2000). Coming, coming, gone: A feminist
deconstruction of heterosexual orgasm. *Sexualities*, 3,
pp. 55–76.

Priest, R. (2001). Missionary Positions: Christian, Modernist,
and Postmodernist. *Current Anthropology*, 42(1), pp. 29–68.

Richters, J et al. (2014). Sex in Australia Summary *2*
[Online] National health and Medical Research Council
Available at: http://www.ashr.edu.au/wp-content/
uploads/2015/06/sex_in_australia_2_summary_data.pdf
[Accessed on 10.09.2019]

Richters, J., de Visser, R., Rissel, C. and Smith, A. (2006). Sexual practices at last heterosexual encounter and occurrence of orgasm in a national survey. *Journal of Sex Research*, 43(3), pp. 217–226.

Rideout, V. J., Foehr, U. G. and Roberts, D. F. (2010). *Generation M2: Media in the Lives of 8- to 18-year Olds.* Menlo Park: Kaiser Family Foundation.

Rider, J. R., Wilson, K. M., Sinnott, J. A., Kelly, J. S., Muccia, L. A. and Giovannucci, E. L. (2016). Ejaculation Frequency and Risk of Prostate Cancer: Updated Results with an Additional Decade of Follow-up. *European Urology*, 70, pp. 974–982.

Rieger, G., Savin-Williams, R.C., Chivers, M. L. and Bailey, J. M. (2016). Sexual arousal and masculinity-femininity of women. *Journal of Personality and Social Psychology*, 111(2), pp. 265–283.

Rogers, C. (1951). *Client-Centered Therapy.* London: Constable.

Roscoe, W. (1998). *Changing Ones: Third and Fourth Genders in Native North America.* New York: Palgrave Macmillan US.

Rosen, R. (2000). Prevalence and risk factors of sexual dysfunction in men and women. *Current Psychiatry Reports*, 2, pp. 189–195.

Ross, Julianne (2015). What the Conversation Around "Yes Means Yes" Is Missing. [Online] Mic. Available at: https://

www.mic.com/articles/114176/what-the-conversation-around-yes-means-yes-is-missing. [Accessed: 7 July 2018]

Rupp, L. (2012). Sexual fluidity "before sex". *Signs,* 37, pp. 849–856.

Rust, P.C.R. (2000). Bisexuality: a contemporary paradox for women. *Journal of Social Issues*, 56(2), pp. 205–221.

Salama, S., Boitrelle, F., Gauquelin, A., Malagrida, L., Thiounn, N. and Desvaux, P. (2015). Nature and origin of "squirting" in female sexuality. *Journal of Sexual Medicine.* 12, pp. 661–666.

Salisbury, C. M. A. and Fisher, W. A. (2014). 'Did You Come?' A Qualitative Exploration of Gender Differences in Beliefs, Experiences, and Concerns Regarding Female Orgasm Occurrence During Heterosexual Sexual Interactions. *Journal of Sex Research,* 51, pp. 616–31.

Sanders, S. A. and Reinisch, J. M. (1999). Would you say you "had sex" if…? *JAMA*, 281, pp. 275–277.

Savin-Williams, R. C. (2017). *Mostly straight: Sexual fluidity among men.* Cambridge, MA: Harvard University Press.

Savin-Williams, R. C., Joyner, K. and Rieger, G. (2012). Prevalence and stability of self-reported sexual orientation identity during young adulthood. *Archives of Sexual Behaviour*, 41, pp. 1–8.

Scutty, S. (2018). At least 8 million IVF babies born in 40 years since historic first. [Online] CNN HealthAvailable at: https://edition.cnn.com/2018/07/03/health/worldwide-ivf-babies-born-study/index.html [Accessed on 24.01.2020]

Seidman, S. (1991). *Romantic longings: Love in America, 1830–1980*. New York: Routledge.

Selterman, D., Garcia, J. R. and Tsapelas, I. (2019). Motivations for Extradyadic Infidelity Revisited. *The Journal of Sex Research*, 56(3), pp. 273–286.

Sharkey, N., van Winsberghe, A., Robbins, S. and Hancock, E. (2017). Our Sexual Future with Robots: A foundation for responsible robotics consultation report. [Online] Responsible Robotics Available at: http://responsible-robotics-myxf6pn3xr.netdna-ssl.com/wp-content/uploads/2017/11/FRR-Consultation-Report-Our-Sexual-Future-with-robots-1-1.pdf [Accessed on 24.01.2020]

Shorter, E. (2005). *Written in the Flesh: A History of Desire*. Toronto: University of Toronto Press.

Simon, W. and Gagnon, J. H. (1999). Sexual scripts. *Culture, Society and Sexuality: A Reader*, eds. R. Parker and P. Aggleton. Philadelphia: UCL Press.

Smith, G., Frankel, S. and Yarnell, J. (1998). Sex and Death: Are They Related? Findings From the Caerphilly Cohort Study. *Journal of Urology*, 160(2), p. 628.

Snowdon, C. T. (1997). 'The "Nature" of Sex Differences: Myths of Male and Female' in: Gowaty P.A. (eds). *Feminism and Evolutionary Biology*. Boston, MA: Springer.

Stewart, D. N. and Szymanski, D. M. (2012). Young Adult Women's Reports of Their Male Romantic Partner's Pornography Use as a Correlate of Their Self-Esteem, Relationship Quality, and Sexual Satisfaction. *Sex Roles*, 67, pp. 257–271.

Szittner, K. (2012). Study exposes secret world of porn addiction. [Online] University of Sydney. Available at: http://sydney.edu.au/news/84.html?newsstoryid=9176 [Accessed on 24.01.2020]

Tannahill, R. (1992). *Sex in History*. London: Scarborough Publishers.

Taylor, T. (1996). *The History of Sex: Four Million Years of Human Sexual Culture*. New York: Bantam Books.

Thorndike, E.L. (1920). A constant error in psychological ratings. *Journal of Applied Psychology*, 4(1), pp. 25–29.

Trivers, R. (1972). *Parental Investment and Sexual Selection*. Chicago: Aldine Publishing Company.

Tsjeng, Z. (2016). Teens these days are queer AF, new study says. [Online] VICE.com Available at: https://www.vice.com/en_us/article/kb4dvz/teens-these-days-are-queer-af-new-study-says [Accessed on 24.01.2020]

Twenge, J., Sherman, R. and Wells, B. (2017). Declines in Sexual Frequency among American Adults, 1989–2014. *Archives of Sexual Behaviour*, 46(8), pp. 2389–2401.

Tyden, T., Olsson, S. and Haggstrom-Nordin, E., (2001). Improved Use of Contraceptives, Attitudes Toward Pornography, and Sexual Harassment Among Female University Students. *Women's Health Issues*, 11(2), pp. 87–94.

Tyson, G., Perta, V.C., Haddadi, H. and Seto, M.C. (2016). A first look at user activity on Tinder. *Advances in Social Networks Analysis and Mining*, pp. 461–466.

van Anders, S. (2012). Testosterone and Sexual Desire in Healthy Women and Men. *Archives of Sexual Behaviour,* 41(6), pp. 1471–1484.

Fernández-Villaverde, J. Greenwood, J. and Guner, N. (2014). From Shame to Game in One Hundred Years: An Economic Model of the Rise in Premarital Sex and its De-Stigmatisation. *Journal of the European Economic Association*, 12(1), pp. 25–61.

Waite, L. and Joyner, K. (2001). Emotional Satisfaction and Physical Pleasure in Sexual Unions: Time Horizon, Sexual Behaviour, and Sexual Exclusivity. *Journal of Marriage and Family,* 63, pp. 247–264.

Weaver J. B., Masland J. L. and Zillmann, D. (1984). Effect of erotica on young men's aesthetic perception of their female sexual partners. *Perceptual and Motor Skills.* 58(3), pp. 929–930.

Weitbrecht, E. M., Whitton, S. W. (2017). Expected, ideal, and actual relational outcomes of emerging adults' "hook-ups". *Personal Relationships*, 24, pp. 902–916.

Wellings, K. (2001). Sexual behaviour in Britain: early heterosexual experience. *Lancet*, 358, pp. 1843–1850.

Wellings, K., Collumbien, M., Slaymaker, E., Singh, S., Hodges, Z., Patel, D. and Bajos, N. (2006). Sexual behaviour in context: a global perspective. *Lancet*, 368(9548), pp. 1706–1728.

Yamamiya, Y., Cash, T. F. and Thompson, J. K. (2006). Sexual Experiences among College Women: The Differential Effects of General Versus Contextual Body Images on Sexuality. *Sex Roles*, 55(5–6), pp. 421–427.

Ybarra, M., Mitchell, K., Hamburger, M., Diener-West, M. and Leaf, P. (2011). X-Rated Material and Perpetration of Sexually Aggressive Behaviour Among Children and Adolescents: Is There a Link? *Aggressive Behaviour*, 37, pp. 1–18.

Yean, C., Benau, E. M., Dakanalis, A., Hormes, J. M., Perone, J. and Timko, C. A. (2013). The relationship of sex and sexual orientation to self-esteem, body shape satisfaction, and eating disorder symptomatology. *Frontiers in Psychology*, (4), p. 887.

YouGov. (2019). Nearly half of Americans say sexuality is a scale. [Online] YouGov. Available at: https://today. yougov.com/topics/lifestyle/articles-reports/2019/06/20/

kinsey-scale-sexuality-millennials-2019-poll [Accessed on: 12.12.2019]

Zentner, M. (2005). Ideal Mate Personality Concepts and Compatibility in Close Relationships: A Longitudinal Analysis. *Journal of Personality and Social Psychology*. 89(2), pp. 242–256.

Zilbergeld, B. (1999). *The New Male Sexuality (Revised edition)*. New York: Bantam Press.

Zillmann D. and Bryant J. (1988). Pornography's impact on sexual satisfaction. *Journal of Applied Social Psychology*, 18(5), pp. 438–453.

Zillmann, D. and Bryant, J. (1988). Effects of Prolonged Consumption of Pornography on Family Values. *Journal of Family Issues*, 9(4), pp. 518–544.

Zsok, F., Haucke, M., De Wit, C.Y. and Barelds, D. P. H. (2017). What kind of love is love at first sight? An empirical investigation. *Personal Relationships*, 24(4), pp. 869–885.

NOTE/DISCLAIMER

Trigger encourages diversity and different viewpoints, however, all views, thoughts, and opinions expressed in this book are the author's own and are not necessarily representative of Trigger as an organisation.

All material in this book is set out in good faith for general guidance and no liability can be accepted for loss or expense incurred in following the information given. In particular this book is not intended to replace expert medical or psychiatric advice. It is intended for informational purposes only and for your own personal use and guidance. It is not intended to diagnose, treat or act as a substitute for professional medical advice.

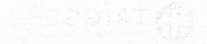

ABOUT TRIGGER PUBLISHING

Trigger is a leading independent altruistic global publisher devoted to opening up conversations about mental health and wellbeing. We share uplifting and inspirational mental health stories, publish advice-driven books by highly qualified clinicians for those in recovery and produce wellbeing books that will help you to live your life with greater meaning and clarity.

Founder Adam Shaw, mental health advocate and philanthropist, established the company with leading psychologist Lauren Callaghan, whilst in recovery from serious mental health issues. Their aim was to publish books which provided advice and support to anyone suffering with mental illness by sharing uplifting and inspiring stories from real-life survivors, combined with expert advice on practical recovery techniques.

Since then, Trigger has expanded to produce books on a wide range of topics surrounding mental health and wellness, as well as launching *Upside Down,* its children's list, which encourages open conversation around mental health from a young age.

We want to help you to not just survive but thrive ... one book at a time.

Find out more about Trigger Publishing by visiting our website:triggerpublishing.com or join us on:

Twitter @TriggerPub
Facebook @TriggerPub
Instagram @TriggerPub

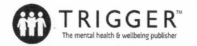

ABOUT SHAW MIND

A proportion of profits from the sale of all Trigger books go to their sister charity, Shaw Mind, also founded by Adam Shaw and Lauren Callaghan. The charity aims to ensure that everyone has access to mental health resources whenever they need them.

You can find out more about the work that Shaw Mind do by visiting their website: shawmindfoundation.org or joining them on
Twitter: @Shaw_Mind
Instagram: @Shaw_Mind
LinkedIn: @shaw-mind
FB: @shawmindUK

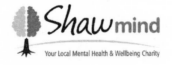

Your Local Mental Health & Wellbeing Charity